CURRENT INSIGHTS IN POLLEN ALLERGENS

Edited by **José C. Jiménez-López**

Current Insights in Pollen Allergens
http://dx.doi.org/10.5772/3312
Edited by José C. Jiménez-López

Contributors

Juan de Dios Alché, Adoración Zafra, Jose Carlos Jiménez-López, Sonia Morales, Antonio Jesús Castro, Fernando Florido, María Isabel Rodríguez-García, Carmen Salmerón, Francisco Manuel Marco, Krzysztof Zienkiewicz, Estefanía García-Quirós, Dieter Volkmann, Toshio Tanaka

Published by InTech

Janeza Trdine 9, 51000 Rijeka, Croatia

Publishing Process Manager Sandra Bakic
Technical Editor InTech DTP team
Cover InTech Design team

Additional hard copies can be obtained from orders@intechopen.com

Current Insights in Pollen Allergens, Edited by José C. Jiménez-López
p. cm.
ISBN 978-953-51-0860-3

For EU product safety concerns:
IN TECH d.o.o., Prolaz Marije Krucifikse Kozulić 3, 51000 Rijeka, Croatia,
info@intechopen.com or visit our website at intechopen.com.

Meet the editor

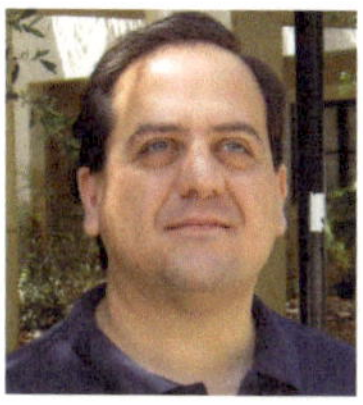

Dr. José C. Jiménez-López graduated in Biochemistry and Molecular Biology (1998), and Biological Sciences (2001) at the University of Granada, Spain. He completed a Masters degree in Agricultural Sciences (2004), and was awarded a PhD degree in 2008 by CSIC. Soon after, he moved to Purdue University (USA) to start with his postdoctoral research in Plant Biology. Finishing this period, in 2011 he was awarded a prestigious Marie Curie Grant to start working in The University of Western Australia. Dr. Jiménez-López has co-authored more than 20 articles in international peer-reviewed journals and 12 book chapters. He has presented his research accomplishments in 45 international conferences, and currently is an active member of six international scientific societies, serving as a referee for several different peer-reviewed journals, and also as a scientific editor for international scientific book editorials as InTech.

Contents

Preface

Pollen allergy is an important public problem and one of the most common causes of chronic ill health in the western societies. More than 25% of the population suffers from IgE-mediated allergies (including children and adults) which therefore represent a major challenge of our society, particularly because untreated allergy often progresses to severe disabling forms of disease. This allergic disease has increased in prevalence during the past decades and a major increase has been predicted.

Today allergen-specific immunotherapy is being established as the only allergen-specific and disease-modifying approach toward the treatment for IgE-mediated allergies and has long lasting effects. Up until now, commonly used treatments have been focused on relief of the clinical symptoms to alleviate allergic inflammation rather than underlying immune mechanisms, i.e. antihistamine and topical corticosteroids. In addition, conventional immunotherapy involves administration of natural allergen extracts containing mixture of undefined components with potential to induce a life-threatening anaphylactic response and new IgE-mediated reactivity and/or sensitizations to previously non-exposes allergens.

At present, there is not universal cure for pollen allergy, and the disease can only be managed by allergens avoidance or treatment of symptoms. However, there is exciting new knowledge as these presented in this book "the cultivar issues", which may help in the improvement of clinical trial, diagnosis and development of potential new therapies.

Researchers in the field are working hard to understand the mechanisms of allergy, and the disease-causing allergens are being characterized in great detail down to their molecular structures and cellular and physiological functions. Advances in molecular biology have led to an exponential increase in our understanding of molecular pathways involved in the manifestation of type 1 allergy symptoms, which also has pave the road for a significant advance in the development of a cure or vaccine for atopic allergic diseases.

Biochemical and molecular approaches together with computational biology, especially the informatics tools for allergen epitopes identification, structural characterization for designing allergy vaccines, have provided the knowledge to resolve structural features of allergen molecules and develop safer form of specific immunotherapy. Various others strategies and approaches are ongoing research programs including cellular and immunological mechanisms of therapy, genetic modification of allergens, hypoallergenic proteins chimera production, DNA vaccines, anti-IgE therapy, different routes of vaccine delivery, reduction of the allergen proteins content in plant-derived food by using RNAi technology, improved production systems for recombinant allergens.

Having this global vision, it seems that we are driving in the right direction to be able developing new and rational forms of diagnosis and therapy strategies. This way holds promise for curing pollen allergy sufferers and eventually may allow real prophylactic vaccination against allergy, i.e. tailored vaccines, or these based in pollen allergen proteins from defined cultivars.

Dr. José C. Jiménez-López
Purdue University,
USA

Pollen Allergenicity is Highly Dependent on the Plant Genetic Background: The "Variety"/"Cultivar" Issues

Juan de Dios Alché, Adoración Zafra, Jose Carlos Jiménez-López, Sonia Morales, Antonio Jesús Castro, Fernando Florido and María Isabel Rodríguez-García

Additional information is available at the end of the chapter

http://dx.doi.org/10.5772/52815

1. Introduction

Type I hypersensibility to pollen is an important cause of allergy worldwide. In other types of allergy like the food allergic symptoms or very frequently the oral allergy syndrome (OAS), clear differences between varieties/cultivars of the same or highly-related plant species have been described as regard to the expression of allergens and their allergenic importance.

Pioneer studies were carried out in date palm tree over the later years of the last century (Kwaasi et al 1999, 2000). Such studies indicated that allergenicity to date fruit was a cultivar-specific phenomenon, and laboratory data showed that individual cultivars varied in their number of IgE immunoblot bands. Sera from fruit-allergic as well as pollen-allergic patients recognized common fruit-specific epitopes. Also, there was heterogeneity in patient responses to the different extracts. Nevertheless, a number of common allergens were responsible for cross-reactivity between the cultivars.

Up to date, similar studies have been carried out in an important number of plants, mainly those producing edible fruits like apple (Asero et al 2006; Rur 2007; Matthes and Schmitz-Eiberger 2009; Vlieg-Boerstra et al 2011), peach (Brenna et al 2004; Ahrazem et al 2007; Chen et al 2008), cherry (Verschuren, http://www.appliedscience.nl/doc/Onderzoek_111117_Martie_Verschuren.pdf), nectarine (Ahrazem et al 2007), tomato (Dölle et al 2011), strawberry (Muñoz et al 2010), and lichy (Hoppe et al 2006) among others, and in seeds like cereals (Nakamura et al 2005), buckwheat (Maruyama-Funatsuki et al 2004) and peanuts (Kang et al 2007; Kottapallia et al 2008).

Numerous analysis have raised the question that pollen grains, similarly to fruits may notably differ among different varieties/cultivars in terms of pollen micromorphology, as well as in their physiological characteristics (e.g. viability, vigour, ability to germinate, compatibility…) (Castro et al 2010; Ribeiro et al 2012), and eventually in their allergenic content. However, literature devoted to the comparison of the pollen allergenic characteristics intra- and inter- varieties is still relatively scarce. This article reviews most of these investigations.

2. Taxonomy of allergenic plants

Excellent reviews have been made as regard to the taxonomical classification of the allergenic plants (Yman1982; Takhtajan 1997; D'Amato et al 1998; Mothes et al 2004; Mohapatra et al 2004; Esch 2004; Radauer et al 2006). Moreover, several broad databases have compiled profuse and well-documented information linking the most relevant plant allergenic sources, the identified allergens and their taxonomical classification. They include Pharmacia (Pharmacia Diagnostics, 2001) and later Phadia/Thermo Fisher Scientific (http://www.phadia.com/en/Allergen-information/ImmunoCAP-Allergens/Allergen-components-list/), the Allergome database of allergenic molecules (Mari et al 2009; http://www.allergome.org/index.php) and the official site for the systematic allergen nomenclature approved by the World Health Organization and International Union of Immunological Societies (WHO/IUIS) Allergen Nomenclature Sub-committee (http://www.allergen.org/index.php). Independently of the widespread presence of cross-reactivity, most allergens are described in these works and databases as characterized in a single species (e.g. rBet v 2 Profilin, Birch= *Betula verrucosa*). Only a minority are referenced to taxonomical entities different to species, either to a combination of related species, cultigens or hybrids (e.g. *Musa acuminata / sapientum / paradisiaca*) or to a heterogeneous group of more than one (often numerous) species (e.g. *Eucalyptus* spp. Note that these abbreviations are not italicized or underlined, and can easily be confused with the abbreviations "ssp." or "subsp." referring to subspecies.). In several cases, allergens are referred to taxonomic ranks of higher entity than species (e.g. *Theaceae*). Only a few allergens are univocally attributed to infraspecific plant categories like varieties (e.g. *Brassica oleraceae var. italica, var. gemmifera, var. capitata, var. botrytis*).

As regards to pollen allergen analysis, two alternatives, apparently opposite, although somehow complementary strategies are defined:

Mothes et al (2004) analyzed cross-reactivities to pollens of trees of the Fagales order, fruits and vegetables, between pollens of the Scrophulariales and pollens of the Coniferales. They proposed a classification of tree pollen and related allergies based on major allergen molecules instead of botanical relationships among the allergenic sources, suggesting Bet v 1 as a marker for Fagales pollen and related plant food allergies, Ole e 1 as a possible marker for Scrophulariales pollen allergy and Cry j 1 and Cry j 2 as potential markers for allergy to Coniferales pollens. Another work analyzed pollen allergen sequences with respect to protein family membership, taxonomic distribution of protein families, and interspecies variability

(Radauer and Breteneder 2006). These authors managed to classify all pollen allergens known to date into a limited number of protein families, and divide them into ubiquitous (e.g. profilins), present in certain families (e.g. pectate lyases), or limited to a single taxon (e.g. thaumatin-like proteins). This approach provides invaluable help in issues like the prediction of cross-reactivity, the design of diagnostic methods and the assessment of the allergenic potential of novel molecules. A similar approach is described by Moreno-Aguilar (2008).

On the other hand, different authors are contributing to define the specific allergenic composition of pollens, going deeper into the taxonomical classification usually observed (this is, characterizing the allergenic composition of pollens at infraspecific level), and abounding into the analysis of pollen allergenic polymorphism. Advantages of such strategy have been outlined before (Alché et al 2007). Diverse examples of this strategy are depicted next.

3. Infraspecific botanical names

In botany, an infraspecific name is that corresponding to any taxon below the rank of species. Such names are constructed based in the use of trinomial nomenclature, regulated by the International Code of Botanical Nomenclature (ICBN) (McNeill et al 2006), which includes: genus name, specific epithet, connecting term indicating the rank (not part of the name, but required), and finally the infraspecific epithet. It is habitual to italicize all three parts of the name, but not the connecting term. Five different taxonomical ranks below the species are explicitly allowed in the ICBN:

a. subspecies - recommended abbreviation: subsp. ("ssp." also widely used)
b. varietas (variety) - recommended abbreviation: var.
c. subvarietas (subvariety) - recommended abbreviation: subvar.
d. forma (form) - recommended abbreviation: f.
e. subforma (subform) - recommended abbreviation: subf.

A **subspecies** is a taxonomical rank formed by individuals of the same species which are capable of interbreeding and producing fertile offspring. However, they often do not interbreed in nature due to geographic isolation or other factors (http://en.wikipedia.org/wiki/Subspecies). The differences between subspecies are usually less distinct than the differences between species, but more distinct than the differences between varieties.

A **botanical variety** is a taxonomic rank below that of species, characterized by differential appearance from other varieties. However, varieties retain the ability to hybridize freely among themselves, providing they become in contact. Usually, varieties are geographically separated. Varieties are named by using the binomial Latin name followed by the term "variety" (usually abbreviated as "var.") and the name of the variety in italics.

Subvarieties, forms and subforms constitute taxonomic ranks of "secondary" importance and are more rarely used. For example, a form usually designates a group with a noticeable but minor deviation. Some botanists believe that there is no need to name forms, since there are theoretically countless numbers of forms based on minor genetic differences (http://en.wikipedia.org/wiki/Form_(botany)).

The term **cultivar** is defined as a plant or group of plants selected for desirable characteristics that can be maintained by propagation (http://en.wikipedia.org/wiki/Cultivar). Most cultivars have been obtained after using agronomical methods, or in some cases, selected from wild populations. Crops and even trees used in forestry are usually cultivars that have been selected for desirable characteristics including improved production, resistance to pests, flavor, timber production etc. Naming of cultivars is recommended by the International Code of Nomenclature for Cultivated Plants (ICNCP) (Brickell et al, 2009), and is formed of the scientific botanical name (Latin) followed by the term "cultivar" (usually abbreviated as "cv.") and a cultivar epithet bounded by single quotation marks, for example: *Olea europaea* cv. 'Picual'.

The terms "cultivar" and "variety" are not equivalent. Although different, both terms are often used as synonyms: thus, "grape varieties" are habitually used in viticulture nomenclature to indicate what should be in reality cultivars, according to the International Code of Nomenclature for Cultivated Plants, since grapes are mostly propagated by cuttings. The same applies to "olive varieties", which should be properly named "olive cultivars". In both, and in many other cases, cuttings are the most frequently selected propagation method, as agronomical, physiological and anatomical properties are not maintained in a stable-manner under sexual reproduction. However, usage of the term variety is well fixed in both viticulture and oliviculture, therefore, a change to the correct term (cultivar) is unlikely to occur.

Finally, the term **cultigen** represents to a plant that has been deliberately altered or selected by humans. It is therefore the result of artificial (anthropogenic) selection. Their naming and origin can be very varied, as it is subjected to different rules and criteria (http://en.wikipedia.org/wiki/Cultigen).

4. Pollens with described differential allergenicity within infraspecific taxonomical ranks

Up to date, the presence of differential allergenicity within infraspecific taxonomical ranks has been demonstrated in the pollen of a significant number of plant species at the allergenic context. Next, we describe pollen allergens in these plants, as well as the most representative literature describing such differences.

4.1. Date palm (*Phoenix dactilifera* L.)

The most relevant allergenic questions regarding this plant are compiled in the following web pages: http://www.phadia.com/en/Allergen-information/ImmunoCAP-Allergens/Food-of-Plant-Origin/Fruits/Date/ (Phadia), and http://www.allergome.org/script/dettaglio.php?id_molecule=1925 (Allergome).

Briefly, *Ph. dactilifera* pollen contains allergens of 14.3 kDa, 27-33 kDa, 54-58 kDa and 90 kDa (Postigo et al 2009). The presence of cross-reactivity among the different individual species of tree pollen of members of the genus could be expected (Yman 1982), and RAST inhibition studies have demonstrated significant cross-reactivity between *P. canariensis* and *P. dactylifera* pollen (Blanco et al 1995).

Kwaasi et al (1994) compared pollen crude extracts from ten cultivars of this tree for their antigenic and allergenic potentials. The results of the tests performed on 6 confirmed atopic patients, including skin prick tests, ELISA, IgG and IgE immunoblotting analyses, peripheral blood lymphocyte proliferation and concomitant interleukin-4 (IL-4) production indicated sharp inter-cultivar heterogeneity. One of the cultivars even failed to elicit any skin test reactivity or bind IgE in atopic sera as determined by the indicated assays. The authors therefore suggest that the antigenicity and allergenicity of date palm pollen is more of a cultivar-specific phenomenon than a species-specific phenomenon, which is governed by the number, quantities or both of the major allergen epitopes possessed by that variety or cultivar. Nevertheless, a number of common allergens are responsible for cross-reactivity between the cultivars.

It has been later demonstrated that antigens and allergens of date fruits cross-react with date pollen allergens and date fruit-sensitive as well as date pollen-allergic patients' sera recognize the same group of date fruit IgE-binding components (Kwaasi et al 1999). Therefore, the cultivar issue is also tremendously important in selecting date cultivars for allergen standardization (Kwaasi et al 2000).

4.2. Arizona cypress (*Cupressus arizonica* L.)

The most relevant allergenic questions regarding this plant are brought together in the following web pages: http://intapp3.phadia.com/en/Allergen-information/ImmunoCAP-Allergens/Tree-Pollens/Allergens/Arizona-cypress-/ (Phadia), and http://www.allergome.org/ script/dettaglio.php?id_molecule=1793 (Allergome).

In brief: *Cupressaceae* pollen is characterized by a low protein concentration and high carbohydrate content. Allergens from the Arizona cypress tree have been isolated, characterized, and their diagnostic significance established (Penon 2000). They include Cup a 1, a 43-kDa protein, characterized as a pectate lyase (Di Felice et al1994; 2001; Afferni et al 1999; Aceituno et al 2000; Alisi et al 2001; Mistrello et al 2002; Iacovacci et al 2002; Arilla et al 2004), rCup a 1 (Aceituno et al 2000; Iacovacci et al 2002), Cup a 2, a polygalacturonase (Di Felice et al 2001; de Coana et al 2006), Cup a 3, a thaumatin-like protein (Cortegano et al 2004; Togawa et al 2006; Suarez-Cervera et al 2008) and Cup a 4, a calcium-binding protein (de Coana 2010). *C. arizonica* and *C. sempervirens* extracts are highly cross-reactive at the IgE level and have a number of common epitopes. Two major IgE-reactive components of approximately 43 kDa and 36 kDa have been shown to be present in both (Barletta et al 1996). *C. sempervirens* shows a wider diversity of allergens, whereas *C. arizonica* shows a higher content of the major 43 kDa allergen (Leduc et al 2000). Extensive cross-reactivity also occurs with other family members, which include *Juniperus oxycedrus*, *Chamaecyparis obtusa* and *Thuja plicata*.

In general, species of the *Cupressaceae* family are a very important cause of allergies in various geographical areas, especially North America, Japan, and Mediterranean countries.

Incidence is growing spectacularly as a consequence of these species been widely used for reforestation, for wind and noise barriers, and ornamentally in gardens and parks, as well as for reforestation (Bousquet et al 1993; Caiaffa et al 1993).

Shahali et al (2007) performed a comparative study of the pollen protein contents in two major varieties of *Cupressus arizonica* (*C. arizonica* var. *arizonica* and *C. arizonica* var. *glabra*) planted in Tehran. Their investigations revealed noticeable differences in protein content of each variety, with a new major protein of c.a. 35 kDa present in the extracts, with high reactivity to the sera from allergic patients. Such band showed even more relevance than the major allergen Cup a 1 (45 kDa), reported as the most representative protein in pollen extracts of Mediterranean countries. Due to the fact that many different Arizona cypress tree varieties exist (recognized on the basis of distribution and of foliage, cone and bark characteristics and furthermore by using RAPDs markers) (Bartel et al 2003), the presence of huge differences in reactivity is expected.

4.3. Birch (*Betula verrucosa*, Synonym: *B. pendula*)

Relevant allergenic information concerning this plant (one of the best characterized allergenic sources up to date) is listed in the next web pages: http://intapp3.phadia.com/en/Allergen-information/ImmunoCAP-Allergens/Tree-Pollens/Allergens/Common-silver-birch-/http://intapp3.phadia.com/en/Allergen-informtion /ImmunoCAP-Allergens/Tree-Pollens/Allergens/Arizona-cypress-/ (Phadia), and http://ww w. allergome.org/script/dettaglio.php?id_molecule=1741 (Allergome).

In short: Birch pollen contains at least 29 antigens (Wiebicke et al 1987). Allergens of molecular weights of 29.5, 17, 12.5, and 13 kDa have been isolated (Florvaag et al 1988; Hirschl, 1989). The following allergens have been characterized: Bet v 1, a 17 kDa protein displaying ribonuclease activity and characterized as a PR-10 protein (Breiteneder et al 1989; Elsayed et al 1990; Grote et al 1993; Scheiner, 1993; Swoboda et al 1994; Taneichi et al 1994; Bufe et al 1996; Holm et al 2001; Mogensen et al 2002; Vieths et al 2002) , Bet v 2, a 15 kDa profilin (Elsayed and Vik, 1990; Valenta et al 1991a,b,c; Grote et al 1993; Scheiner, 1993; Seiberler et al 1994; Wiedemann et al 1996; Engel et al 1997; Domke et al 1997; Fedorov et al 1997; Vieths et al 2002), Bet v 3, a 24 kDa calcium-binding protein (Seiberler et a. 1994; Tinghino et al 2002). Bet v 4, a 9 kDa Ca-binding protein (Engel et al 1997; Twardosz et al 1997; Ferreira et al 1999; Grote et al 2002), Bet v 5, a 35 kDa isoflavone reductase-related protein (Vieths et al 1998; Karamloo et al 1999; Stewart and McWilliam, 2001), Bet v 6, a 30-35 kDa protein, PCBER (Phenylcoumaran benzylic ether reductase) (Karamloo et al 2001), Bet v 7, a 18 kDa protein, characterized as a cyclophilin (Cadot et al 2000) and Bet v 11 (Moverare et al 2002).

A large number of these allergens have been expressed as recombinant proteins, including rBet v 1 (Ferreira et al 2003), rBet v 2 (Valenta et al 1991a-c; Niederberger et al 1998; Susani et al 1995; Valenta et al 1993), rBet v 3 (Valenta et al 1991a-c; Seiberler et al 1994), rBet v 4 (Engel et al 1997; Twardosz et al 1997; Ferreira et al 1999), rBet v 5 (Karamloo et al 1999) and rBet v 6 (Vieths et al 2002).

As significant allergenic behaviors, Bet v 1 displays a considerable degree of heterogeneity and consists of at least 20 isoforms which differ in their IgE-binding capacity (Bet v 1a to Bet v 1n), (Breiteneder et al 1989; Elsayed and Vik, 1990; Karamloo et al 1999; Friedl-Hajek et al 1999). Birch pollen-allergic individuals may not be sensitized to any of the major birch pollen allergens.

Evidence of cross-reactivity of birch allergens among different sources is very high: Cross-reactivity exists between pollens from species within the *Betulaceae* family or belonging to closely related families (Valenta et al 1991a-c, 1993; Yman 1982, 2001; Eriksson et al 1987; Jung et al 1987; Ipsen et al 1985; Breiteneder et al 1993; Kos et al 1993; Wahl et al 1996). Moreover, the presence of numerous so-called cross reactivity syndrome have been described, including the "Birch-Mugwort-Celery syndrome" (Ballmer-Weber et al 2000) and the "Celery-Carrot-Birch-Mugwort-spice syndrome" when Carrot and Spices are included (Pauli et al 1985; Dietschi et al 1987; Helbling 1997; Wüthrich and Dietschi 1985; Stäger et al 1991). The major birch pollen allergen, Bet v 1, and the apple allergen Mald 1 share allergic epitopes leading to IgE cross-reactivities (Ebner et al 1991; Vieths et al 1994; Matthes and Schmitz-Eiberger 2009). Especially during the birch pollen season, an increase in clinical reactions to apples occurs (Skamstrup-Hansen et al 2001). The most common manifestation of allergy to food in Birch pollen-allergic individuals is oral allergy syndrome (OAS).

Selection and breeding of hypoallergenic trees or the application of genetic modification to develop these may potentially reduce the allergenic load caused by birch. This and other objectives have led to the development of studies to characterize genes encoding Bet v 1 isoforms (Schenk et al 2006, 2009). Such studies included the screening of different *Betula* species and different *Betula pendula* cultivars. In total, fourteen different Bet v I-type isoforms were identified in three cultivars, of which nine isoforms were entirely new (Schenk et al 2006). A major conclusion of this study is that a single birch tree may produce a mixture of isoforms with varying IgE reactivity, and that this fact should be taken into account in investigations towards sensitization and immunotherapy. Variability of Bet v I and closely related PR-10 genes in the genome was established by Schenk et al (2009) in eight birch species including *B. pendula* and a particular *B. pendula* cultivar named 'Youngii'. Expression studies of these genes were also carried out by using Q-TOF LC-MS^E methods.

A recent publication by Schenk et al (2011) analyzes antigenic and allergenic profiles of pollen extracts from several genotypes of birch species, including several hybrids, and four cultivars of *Betula pendula* by SDS-PAGE and Western blot using pooled sera of birch-allergic individuals. Tryptic digests of the Bet v 1 were subjected to LC-MS^E analysis. Considerable differences in Bet v 1 isoform composition exist between birch genotypes.

Schenk et al (2008) reviewed the controversial taxonomy of *Betula*, and the various classifications historically proposed. The basic chromosome number of *Betula* is $n=14$, and the species form a series of polyploids with chromosome numbers of $2n=28$, 56, 70, 84, 112, and 140. Moreover, several of the recognized *Betula* species have a hybrid origin. The simultaneous occurrence of polyploidization, extensive hybridization, and introgression complicates even more taxonomical studies in the genus. These authors also reviewed the different methods and alternative markers (including DNA markers) used to reconstruct species relationships within the genus *Betula*. The authors examined the use of AFLPs for this purpose in 107 *Betula* accessions from 23 species and 11 hybrids. At least 9 well determined subspecies, varieties, or cultivars of *Betula pendula* were included in this study along another 24 infraspecies-undetermined accessions of this species. This gives an idea of the wide germplasm involved, and the difficulty of characterizing the different allergenic variants present in the corresponding pollen.

4.4. Japanese cedar (*Cryptomeria japonica*, Synonym: *Cupressus japonica*)

Relevant allergenic information concerning this plant is assembled in the web pages http://www.phadia.com/en/Allergen-information/ImmunoCAP-Allergens/Tree-Pollens/Allergens/Japanese-cedar-/ (Phadia), and http://www.allergome.org/script/dettaglio.php?id_molecule=1784 (Allergome).

The following allergens have been characterized in this source: Cry j 1, a 45-50 kDa protein, a pectate lyase, is considered a major allergen (Yasueda et al 1983; Taniai et al 1988; Griffith et al 1993; Sone et al 1994; Taniguchi et al 1995; Hashimoto et al 1995; Okano et al 2001; Goto et al 2004; Okano et al 2004; Maeda et al 2005;Takahashi et al 2006; Midoro-Horiuti et al 2006; Kimura et al 2008), Cry j 2, a polygalacturonase, also considered a major allergen (Sakaguchi et al 1990; Namba et al 1994; Komiyama et al 1994; Taniguchi et al 1995; Ohtsuki et al 1995; Futamura et al 2006; Goto-Fukuda et al 2007), Cry j 3, a 27 kDa protein characterized as a thaumatin, and a PR-5 protein (Fujimura et al 2007; Futamura et al 2002, 2006), Cry j 4, a Ca-binding protein (Futamura et al 2006), Cry j IFR, an isoflavone reductase (Kawamoto et al 2002), Cry j, a chitinase (Fujimura et al 2005), Cry j AP, a Aspartic Protease (Ibrahim et al 2010a), Cry j CPA9, a serin protease (Ibrahim et al 2010b), and Cry j LTP, a Lipid Transfer Protein (Ibrahim et al 2010c). Moreover, a number of other antigenic proteins have been isolated but not characterized, including proteins of 7, 15 and 20 kDa (Matsumura et al 2006).

Cross-reactivity among conifer pollens has been documented (Aceituno et al 2000; Midoro-Horiuti et al 1999; Ito et al 1995). This could be explained by the high similarity between the Japanese cedar allergen Cry j 1 and the major allergens of Mountain cedar (Jun a 1), Japanese cypress (Cha o 1) and *Cupressus arizonica* (Cup a 1). Other cross-reactivities include tomato fruit (Kondo et al 2002), latex (Fujimura 2005) and *Cupressus sempervirens* (Panzani et al 1986).

Cry j 1 and Cry j 2 are major allergens. However, concentrations of these allergens vary greatly in pollen from different individual Japanese cedar trees (Goto-Fukuda et al 2007). Most basically, there are 2 varieties of Japanese cedar trees: the popular diploid and the less popular triploid. These trees are not very different morphologically. In a comparison of the major allergens Cry j 1 and Cry j 2, the triploid tree pollen extract was shown to have lower concentrations of both. The pollen from this variety may thus be less allergenic (Kondo et al 1997). Conspicuous differences were detected in the presence of the Cry j 1 allergen in two kinds of cultivar: 'Mio' and 'Masuyama' (Saito and Teranishi, 2002).

4.5. Olive tree (*Olea europaea* L.)

Relevant allergenic information concerning this plant is compiled in the web pages http://www.phadia.com/en/Allergen-information/ImmunoCAP-Allergens/Tree-Pollens/Allergens/Olive-/(Phadia), and http://www.allergome.org/script/dettaglio.php?id_molecule=1888 (Allergome). Furthermore, a very recent article by Esteve et al (2012) reviews the information available about the characterized olive allergens at present, the procedures used for such physicochemical and immunological characterization, as well as for extraction and production of olive allergens. Up to date, twelve allergens have been identified in olive pollen while just one allergen has been identified in olive fruit. Additional reviews on olive pollen allergens include the chapters by Jimenez-Lopez et al, Morales et al, and Zienkiewicz et al included in this book.

Olive pollen is by far the most studied allergenic pollen at infraspecific taxonomical level. An important point to explain this is the fact that the olive germplasm (extremely rich although still unexplored in its totality), is the subject of numerous analysis carried out in order to characterize cultivar identity. These works include the use of morphological traits (Barranco and Rallo, 1984; Cimato et al, 1993; Barranco et al, 2005; Caballero et al, 2006) as well as molecular methods, which started with the use of isoenzyme markers (Ouazzani et al, 1993; Trujillo et al, 1995) and at a later stage have been carried out utilizing DNA markers as RFLPs (Besnard et al 2001), RAPDs (Belaj et al, 2001; Fabbri et al, 1995), AFLPs (Angiolillo et al, 1999) and microsatellite markers (SSRs). SSRs are one of the most reliable methods used in olive cultivar characterization (Baldoni et al, 2009; La Mantia et al, 2005). SSRs markers have been successfully used in germplasm bank classification and contributed to a better management of several olive collections around the world (Khadari et al, 2003; Muzzalupo et al, 2006; Fendri et al 2010). In order to provide a better world-wide applicable tool for olive DNA typing, a list of 11 SSRs markers has been selected among microsatellites available for olive cultivar characterization (Baldoni et al, 2009). These works have led to the publication of different olive cultivar catalogues (Barranco and Rallo 1984; Cimato et al 1993; Barranco et al 2000; Caballero et al 2006).

Earlier evidence of the relationships between olive allergen polymorphism and the cultivar origin of olive pollen was reviewed by Alché et al (2007), with particular reference to the publications available at that time, including those by Barber et al 1990, Geller-Bernstein et al (1996), Waisel and Geller-Bernstein (1996), Castro (2001, 2003), Carnes Sanchez et al (2002), Conde Hernandez et al (2002), Hamman-Khalifa et al (2003, 2005), Alché et al (2003), Napoli et al (2006) and Fernandez-Caldas et al (2007). Further confirmation at the molecular level has risen since, based in the use of powerful cloning, proteomics (peptide mapping and N-glycopeptide analysis) and bioinformatics methods. These include the analysis of numerous cDNA and peptide/glucan sequences from Ole e 1 (Napoli et al, 2008; Hamman Khalifa et al, 2010; Castro et al, 2012; Jiménez-López et al, 2011; Soleimani et al, 2012a,b), Ole e 5 (Zafra, 2007), Ole e 2 (Jiménez López, 2008; Morales et al, 2008; Jiménez-López et al, 2012b), and Ole e 11 (Jiménez-López et al, 2012a). Moreover, the reactivity of a broad panel of olive pollen cultivar extracts to diverse patient' sera has been also analyzed in Jordan (Jaradat et al, 2011). Recently, a novel multiplex method for the simultaneous detection and relative quantification of pollen allergens has been set up (Morales 2012; Morales et al, 2012). This method will help to investigate pollen allergen polymorphism within cultivars in combination with patient's reactivity, by notably improving the specificity and capacity of the biochemical and immunological assays. The present book also includes remarkable analyses of olive varietal polymorphism in those chapters by Jimenez-Lopez et al, Morales et al, and Zienkiewicz et al

5. Conclusions and future perspectives

The past and recent developments in the analysis of the differential allergenicity of pollens from heterogeneous infraspecific taxonomic ranks described above, confirm the need of rethinking current strategies for basic research on pollen allergen characterization, and the design of diagnosis and specific immunotherapy approaches. These issues, raised and discussed initially by us (Alché et al, 2007) for olive pollen allergens, seem to be valid for a broader number of species, as stated here. Extensive pollen allergen polymorphism is known to represent a general feature over the plant kingdom. The limitation of the study of this polymorphism just to the level of species represents a restriction which may limit both basic knowledge and more importantly the efficacy and the future development of strategies to detect and contest human pollen allergy. Although the use of marker allergens for order, genera or even plant families may represent an invaluable tool (Mothes et al, 2004), relevant differences in patient's reactivity occur even among close-related taxonomical ranks (e.g. van Ree 2002; Asero et al, 2005; Fenaille et al, 2009; Wallner et al, 2009a,b; Jaradat et al, 2011) therefore determining that even close allergenic compositions are not always "fully equivalent". The analysis of allergenic variability in infraspecific taxonomical ranks should be considered a "must" that can be easily incorporated into most developing and evolving trends in allergy analysis and clinics, namely the design of highly specific and personalized natural extracts, hypoallergens, the design and production of recombinant allergens, hybrid molecules, high-throughput diagnosis, new forms of allergen administration and release, the analysis of allergen cross-reactivity etc. (Schenk et al, 2006, 2011; Gao et al, 2008; Wallner et al, 2009a,b).

Agricultural and environmental strategies to reduce the impact of pollen allergy involving the use of differential infraspecific taxonomic ranks are not to be discarded either. They may include the primary screening of relatively less allergenic varieties as proposed for wheat, buckwheat and other food sources (Nair and Adachi, 2002; Nakamura et al, 2005; Spangenberg et al, 2006), and the future design of varieties/hybrids with reduced pollen production, limited period of flowering, or even androsteril characteristics in a similar way of that proposed for the Gilissen et al (2006a,b) for the production of hypoallergenic plant foods by selection, breeding and genetic modifications.

Author details

Juan de Dios Alché*, Adoración Zafra, Jose Carlos Jiménez-López,
Antonio Jesús Castro and María Isabel Rodríguez-García
Department of Biochemistry, Cell and Molecular Biology of Plants, Estación Experimental del Zaidín, Consejo Superior de Investigaciones Científicas (CSIC), Granada, Spain

Sonia Morales
Department of Biochemistry, Cell and Molecular Biology of Plants, Estación Experimental del Zaidín, Consejo Superior de Investigaciones Científicas (CSIC), Granada, Spain
Proteomic Research Service, Hospital Universitario San Cecilio, Granada, Spain

Fernando Florido
Allergy Service, Hospital Universitario San Cecilio, Granada, Spain

Acknowledgement

This work was funded by ERDF (co)-financed projects P2010-CVI5767, P2010-AGR6274, BFU2011-22779, P2011-CVI-7487 and PEOPLE-IOF/1526.

6. References

Aceituno, E., Del Pozo, V., Mínguez, A., Arrieta, I., Cortegano, I., Cárdaba, B., Gallardo, S., Rojo, M., Palomino, P. & Lahoz, C. (2000). Molecular cloning of major allergen from *Cupressus arizonica* pollen: Cup a 1. *Clinical and Experimental Allergy*, Vol. 30, No. 12, pp. 1750-1758.

Afferni, C., Iacovacci, P., Barletta, B., Di Felice, G., Tinghino, R., Mari, A. & Pini, C. (1999). Role of carbohydrate moieties in IgE binding to allergenic components of *Cupressus arizonica* pollen extract. *Clinical and Experimental Allergy*, Vol. 29, No. 8, pp. 1087-1094.

Ahrazem, O., Jimeno, L., López-Torrejón, G., Herrero, M., Espada, J.L., Sánchez-Monge, R., Duffort, O., Barber, D. & Salcedo, G. (2007). Assessing allergen levels in peach and nectarine cultivars. *Annals of Allergy, Asthma & Immunology*, Vol, 99, No. 1, pp. 42-47.

Alché, J.D., Castro, A.J., Jiménez-López, J.C., Morales, S., Zafra, A., Hamman-Khalifa, A.M., & Rodríguez-García, M.I. (2007). Differential characteristics of the olive pollen from different cultivars and its biological and clinical implications. *Journal of Investigational Allergology & Clinical Immunology*, Vol. 17, Suppl 1., pp. 63-68.

Alisi, C., Afferni, C., Iacovacci, P., Barletta, B., Tinghino, R., Butteroni, C., Puggioni, E.M., Wilson, I.B., Federico, R., Schininà, M.E., Ariano, R., Di Felice, G. & Pini, C. (2001).

* Corresponding Author

Rapid isolation, characterization, and glycan analysis of Cup a 1, the major allergen of Arizona cypress (*Cupressus arizonica*) pollen. *Allergy*, Vol. 56, No. 10, pp. 978-984.

Angiolillo, A., Mencuccini, M. & L. Baldoni, L. (1999). Olive genetic diversity assessed using amplified fragment length polymorphisms. *Theoretical and Applied Genetics*, Vol. 98, No. 3-4, pp. 411-421.

Arilla, M.C., Ibarrola, I., Garcia, R., De La Hoz, B., Martinez, A. & Asturias, J.A. (2004). Quantification of the Major Allergen from Cypress (*Cupressus arizonica*) Pollen, Cup a 1, by Monoclonal Antibody-Based ELISA. *International Archives of Allergy and Immunology*, Vol. 134, No.1, pp. 10-16.

Asero, R., Marzban, G., Martinelli, A., Zaccarini, M. & Machado, M.L. (2006). Search for low-allergenic apple cultivars for birch-pollen-allergic patients: is there a correlation between in vitro assays and patient response? *European Annals of Allergy and Clinical Immunology*, Vol. 38, No. 3, pp. 94-8.

Asero, R., Weber, B., Mistrello, G., Amato, S., Madonini, E. & Cromwell, O. (2005). Giant ragweed specific immunotherapy is not effective in a proportion of patients sensitized to short ragweed: Analysis of the allergenic differences between short and giant ragweed. *Journal of Allergy and Clinical Immunology*, Vol. 116, No. 5, pp. 1036–1041.

Baldoni, L., Cultrera, N.G., Mariotti, R., Ricciolini, C., Arcioni, S., Vendramin, G.G, Buonamici, A., Porceddu, A., Sarri, V., Ojeda, M.A., Trujillo, I., Rallo, L., Belaj, A., Perri, E., Salimonti, A., Muzzalupo, I., Casagrande, A., Lain, O., Messina, R. & Testolin, R. (2009). A consensus list of microsatellite markers for olive genotyping. *Molecular Breeding*, Vol. 24, No. 3, pp. 213-231.

Ballmer-Weber, B.K., Vieths, S., Luttkopf, D., Heuschmann, P. & Wüthrich, B. (2000). Celery allergy confirmed by double-blind, placebo-controlled food challenge: a clinical study in 32 subjects with a history of adverse reactions to celery root. *The Journal of Allergy and Clinical Immunology*, Vol. 106, No. 2, pp. 373-378.

Barletta, B., Afferni, C., Tinghino, R., Mari, A., Di Felice, G. & Pini, C. (1996). Cross-reactivity between *Cupressus arizonica* and *Cupressus sempervirens* pollen extracts. *The Journal of Allergy and Clinical Immunology*, Vol. 98, No. 4, pp. 797-804.

Barranco, D., & L. Rallo. (1984). Las variedades de olivo cultivadas en Andalucía. *Ministerio de Agricultura. Junta de Andalucía*. Madrid. Spain.

Barranco, D., A. Cimato, P., Fiorino, L., Rallo, A., Touzani, C., Castañeda, F., Serafín & Trujillo, I. (2000). *World catalogue of olive varieties. Internacional Olive Oil Council*. Madrid. España.

Barranco, D., Trujillo, I., & L. Rallo, L. (2005). Libro I Elaiografía Hispánica. L. Rallo, D. Barranco, J.M. Caballero, C. Del Rio, A. Martin, J. Tous, and I. Trujillo (eds). *Variedades de olivo en España. Junta de Andalucía, MAPA y Ediciones Mundi-Prensa, Madrid,* pp. 45-231.

Bartel, J.A., Adams, R.P., James, S.A., Mumba, L.E. & Pandey, R.N. (2003). Variation among Cupressus species from the western hemisphere based on random amplified polymorphic DNAs. *Biochemical Systematics and Ecology*, Vol. 31, 693–702.

Belaj, A., Trujillo, I., de la Rosa, R., Rallo, L. & Giménez, M.J. (2001). Polymorphism and discriminating capacity of randomly amplified polymorphic markers in an olive germplasm bank. *Journal of the American Society for Horticultural Science*, Vol. 126, No. 1, pp. 64-71.

Besnard, G., Batadat, P., Chevalier, D., Tagmount, A. & Bervillé, A. (2001). Genetic differentiation in the olive complex (*Olea europaea*) revealed by RAPDs and RFLPs in the rRNA genes. *Genetic Resources and Crop Evolution*, Vol. 48, pp. 165-182.

Blanco, C., Carrillo, T., Quiralte, J., Pascual, C., Martin Esteban, M. & Castillo, R. (1995). Occupational rhinoconjunctivitis and bronchial asthma due to *Phoenix canariensis* pollen allergy. *Allergy*, Vol. 50, No. 3, pp. 277-80.

Bousquet, J., Knani, J., Hejjaoui, A., Ferrando, R., Cour, P., Dhivert, H. & Michel, F.B. (1993). Heterogeneity of atopy. I. Clinical and immunologic characteristics of patients allergic to cypress pollen. *Allergy*, Vol. 48, No.3, pp. 183-188.

Breiteneder, H., Ferreira, F., Hoffmann-Sommergruber, K., Ebner, C., Breitenbach, M., Rumpold, H., Kraft, D. & Scheiner, O. (1993). Four recombinant isoforms of Cor a I, the major allergen of hazel pollen, show different IgE-binding properties. *European Journal of Biochemistry*, Vol. 212, No. 2, pp. 355-362.

Breiteneder, H., Pettenburger, K., Bito, A., Valenta, R., Kraft, D., Rumpold, H., Scheiner, O. & Breitenbach, M. (1989). The gene encoding for the major birch pollen allergen Bet v 1 is highly homologous to a pea disease resistance response gene. *The EMBO Journal*, Vol. 8, No. 7, pp. 1935-1938.

Brenna, O.V., Pastorello, E.A., Farioli, L., Pravettoni, V. & Pompei, C. (2004). Presence of allergenic proteins in different peach (*Prunus persica*) cultivars and dependence of their content on fruit ripening. *Journal of Agricultural and Food Chemistry*, Vol. 52, No. 26, pp. 7997-8000.

Brickell, C.D., Alexander, C., David, J.C., Hetterscheid, W.L.A., Leslie, A.C., Malecot, V., Xiaobai Jin, & Cubey, J.J. (2009). International code of nomenclature for cultivated plants. *International Society for Horticultural Science*, Scripta Horticulturae 10, 204 pages.

Bufe, A., Spangfort, M.D., Kahlert, H., Schlaak, M. & Becker, W.M. (1996). The major birch pollen allergen, Bet v 1, shows ribonuclease activity. *Planta*, Vol. 199, No. 3, pp. 413-415.

Caballero, J.M., del Rio, C., Barranco, D., & Trujillo, I. (2006). The Olive World Germplasm Bank of Córdoba, Spain. *Olea*, Vol. 25, pp. 14-19.

Cadot, P., Diaz, J.F., Proost, P., Van D.J., Engelborghs, Y., Stevens, E.A. & Ceuppens, J.L. (2000). Purification and characterization of an 18-kd allergen of birch (*Betula verrucosa*) pollen: identification as a cyclophilin. *The Journal of Allergy and Clinical Immunology*, Vol. 105, No. 2 (Pt1), pp. 286-291.

Caiaffa, M.F., Macchia, L., Strada, S., Bariletto, G., Scarpelli, F. & Tursi, A. (1993). Airborne Cupressaceae pollen in southern Italy. *Annals of Allergy*, Vol. 71, No. 1, pp. 45-50.

Carnés Sánchez, J., Iraola, V.M., Sastre, J., Florido, F., Boluda, L. & Fernandez-Caldas, E. (2002). Allergenicity and immunochemical characterization of six varieties of Olea europaea. *Allergy*, Vol. 57, No. 4, pp 313-318.

Castro, A.J. (2001). Aproximación a la función biológica del alérgeno mayoritario del polen del olivo (Ole e 1). Implicaciones clínicas y ambientales. Doctoral thesis. Granada (Spain): University of Granada.

Castro, A.J., Alché, J.D., Cuevas, J., Romero, P.J., Alché, V. & Rodríguez-García, M.I. (2003). Pollen from different olive tree cultivars contains varying amounts of the major allergen Ole e 1. *International Archives of Allergy and Immunology*, Vol. 131, NO. 3, pp. 164-173.

Castro, A.J., Bednarczyk, A., Schaeffer-Reiss, C., Rodríguez-García, M.I., Van Dorsselaer, A. & Alché, J.D. (2010). Screening of Ole e 1 polymorphism among olive cultivars by peptide mapping and N-glycopeptide analysis. *Proteomics*, Vol. 10, No. 5, pp. 953-621.

Castro, A.J., Rejón, J.D., Fendri, M., Jiménez-Quesada, M.J., Zafra, A., Jiménez-López, J.C., Rodríguez-García, M.I. & Alché, J.D. (2010). Taxonomical discrimination of pollen grains by using confocal laser scanning microscopy (CLSM) imaging of autofluorescence. *Microscopy: Science, Technology, Applications and Education. FORMATEX Microscopy Series Nº 4*, Vol. 4, pp. 607-613.

Chen, L., Zhang, S., Illa, E., Song, L., Wu, S., Howad, W., Arús, P., Weg, E., Chen K. & Gao, Z. (2008). Genomic characterization of putative allergen genes in peach/almond and their synteny with apple. *BMC Genomics*, Vol, 9, p. 543.

Cimato, A., Cantini, C., Sani, G. & Marranci, M. (1993). II Germoplasma dell' Olivo in Toscana. Ed. *Regione Toscana*, Florence, Italy. p. 1254.

Conde Hernández, J., Conde Hernández, P., González Quevedo Tejerina, M.T., Conde Alcañiz, M.A., Conde Alcañiz, E.M., Crespo Moreira, P. & Cabanillas Platero, M. Antigenic and allergenic differences between 16 different cultivars of Olea europaea. *Allergy*, Vol. 57, Suppl. 71, pp. 60-65.

Cortegano, I., Civantos, E., Aceituno, E., Del Moral, A., Lopez, E., Lombardero, M., Del Pozo, V., Lahoz, C. (2004). Cloning and expression of a major allergen from *Cupressus arizonica* pollen, Cup a 3, a PR-5 protein expressed under polluted environment. *Acta Allergologica*, Vol. 59, No. 5, pp. 485-490.

D'Amato, G., Spieksma, F.T., Liccardi, G., Jäger, S., Russo, M., Kontou-Fili, K., Nikkels, H., Wüthrich, B & Bonini, S. (1998). Pollen-related allergy in Europe. *Allergy*, Vol. 53, No. 6, pp. 567-578.

de Coana, Y.P., Parody, N., Fuertes, M.A., Carnes, J., Roncarolo, D., Ariano, R., Sastre, J., Mistrello, G. & Alonso, C. (2010). Molecular cloning and characterization of Cup a 4, a new allergen from *Cupressus arizonica*. *Biochemical and Biophysical Research Communications*, Vol. 401, No. 3, pp. 451-457.

Di Felice, G., Barletta, B., Tinghino, R. & Pini, C. (2001) Cupressaceae pollinosis: identification, purification and cloning of relevant allergens. *International Archives of Allergy and Immunology*, Vol. 125, No. 4, pp.280-289.

Di Felice, G., Caiaffa, M.F., Bariletto, G., Afferni, C., Di Paolab, R., Mari, A., Palumbo, S., Tinghino, R., Sallusto, F., Tursi, A., Macchia, L., Pini, C. (1994). Allergens of Arizona cypress (*Cupressus arizonica*) pollen: characterization of the pollen extract and identification of the allergenic components. *The Journal of Allergy and Clinical Immunology*, Vol. 94, No. 3 (Pt 1), pp. 547-555.

Dietschi, R., Wüthrich, B. & Johansson, S.G.O. (1987). So-called "celery-carrot-mugwort-spice syndrome." RAST results with new spice discs. *Schweiz Med Wochenschr*, Vol. 87, No. 62, pp.524-531.

Dölle, S., Lehmann, K., Schwarz, D., Weckwert, W., Scheler, C., George, E., Franken, P. & Worm, M. (2011). Allergenic activity of different tomato cultivars in tomato allergic subjects. *Clinical and Experimental Allergy,* Vol. 41, No. 11, pp. 1643-1652.

Domke, T., Federau, T., Schluter, K., Giehl, K., Valenta, R., Schomburg, D. & Jockusch, B.M. (1997). Birch pollen profilin: structural organization and interaction with poly-(L-proline) peptides as revealed by NMR. *FEBS Letters,* Vol. 411, No. 2-3, pp. 291-295.

Ebner, C., Birkner, T., Valenta, R., Rumpold, H., Breitenbach, M., Scheiner, O. & Kraft, D. (1991). Common epitopes of birch pollen and apples-studies by western and northern blot. *The Journal of Allergy and Clinical Immunology,* Vol. 88, No. 4, pp. 588– 594.

Elsayed, S & Vik, H. (1990). Purification and N-terminal amino acid sequence of two birch pollen isoallergens (Bet v I and Bet v II). *International Archives of Allergy and Applied Immunology,* Vol. 93, No. 4, pp. 378-384.

Engel, E., Richter, K., Obermeyer, G., Briza, P., Kungl, A.J., Simon, B., Auer, M., Ebner, C., Rheinberger, H.J., Breitenbach, M. & Ferreira, F. (1997). Immunological and biological properties of Bet v 4, a novel birch pollen allergen with two EF-hand calcium binding domains. *The Journal of Biological Chemistry,* Vol. 272, No. 45, pp. 28630-28637.

Eriksson, N.E., Wihl, J.A., Arrendal, H. & Strandhede, S.O. Tree pollen allergy. III. (1987). Cross reactions based on results from skin prick tests and the RAST in hay fever patients. A multi-centre study. *Allergy,* Vol. 42, No. 3, pp. 205-214.

Esch, R.E. (2004). Grass pollen allergens. Allergens and Allergen Immunotherapy. *Marcel Dekker, Inc. New York,* pp. 185-206.

Esteve, C., Montealegre, C., Marina, M.L. & García, M.C. (2012). Analysis of olive allergens. *Talanta,* Vol. 15, No. 92, pp. 1-14.

Fabbri, A., Hormaza, J.I. & Polito V.S. (1995). Random amplified polymorphic DNA analysis of olive (*Olea europaea* L.) cultivars. *Journal of the American Society for Horticultural Science,* Vol. 120, No.1, pp. 538-542.

Fedorov, A.A., Ball, T., Valenta, R. & Almo, S.C. (1997). X-ray crystal structures of birch pollen profilin and Phl p 2. *International Archives of Allergy and Immunology,* Vol. 113, No, 1-3, pp.109-113.

Fenaille, F., Nony, E., Chabre, H., Lautrette, A., Couret, M.N., Batard, T., Moingeon, P. & Ezan E. (2009). Mass spectrometric investigation of molecular variability of grass pollen group 1 allergens. *Journal of Proteome Research,* Vol. 8, No. 8, pp. 4014-4027.

Fendri, M., Trujillo, M., Trigui, A., Rodríguez-García, M.I. & Alché J.D. (2010). Simple sequence repeat identification and endocarp characterization of olive tree accessions in a Tunisian germplasm collection. *HortScience,*Vol. 45, No. 10, pp. 1429-1436.

Fernández-Caldas, E., Carnés, J., Iraola, V. & Casanovas, M. (2007). Comparison of the allergenicity and Ole e 1 content of 6 varieties of *Olea euroapea* pollen collected during 5 consecutive years. *Annals of Allergy, Asthma & Immunology,* Vol. 98, No. 5, pp. 464-470.

Ferreira, F., Engel, E., Briza, P., Richter, K., Ebner, C. & Breitenbach, M. (1999). Characterization of recombinant Bet v 4, a birch pollen allergen with two EF-hand calcium-binding domains. *International Archives of Allergy and Immunology,* Vol. 118, No. 2-4, pp. 304-305.

Ferreira, F.D., Hoffmann-Sommergruber, K., Breiteneder, H., Pettenburger, K., Ebner, C., Sommergruber, W., Steiner, R., Bohle, B., Sperr, W.R., Valent, P., Kungl, A. J., Breitenbach, M., Kraft, D., & Scheiner, O. (1993). Purification and characterization of recombinant Bet v I, the major birch pollen allergen. Immunological equivalence to natural Bet v I. *The Journal of Biological Chemistry*, Vol. 68, No. 26, pp. 19574-1980.

Florvaag, E., Holen, E., Vik, H. & Elsayed, S. (1988). Comparative studies on tree pollen allergens. XIV. Characterization of the birch (*Betula verrucosa*) and hazel (*Corylus avellana*) pollen extracts by horizontal 2-D SDS-PAGE combined with electrophoretic transfer and IgE immunoautoradiography. *Annals of Allergy*, Vol. 61, No. 5, pp. 392-400.

Friedl-Hajek, R., Radauer, C., O'Riordain, G., Hoffmann-Sommergruber, K., Leberl, K., Scheiner, O. & Breiteneder, H. (1999). New Bet v 1 isoforms including a naturally occurring truncated form of the protein derived from Austrian birch pollen. *Molecular Immunology*, Vol. 36, No. 10, pp. 639-645.

Fujimura, T., Shigeta, S., Suwa, T., Kawamoto, S., Aki, T., Masubuchi, M., Hayashi, T., Hide, M. & Ono, K. (2005). Molecular cloning of a class IV chitinase allergen from Japanese cedar (Cryptomeria japonica) pollen and competitive inhibition of its immunoglobulin E-binding capacity by latex C-serum. *Clinical and Experimental Allergy*, Vol. 35, No. 2, pp. 234-243.

Fujimura, T., Futamura, N., Midoro-Horiuti, T., Togawa, A., Goldblum, R.M., Yasueda, H., Saito, A., Shinohara, K., Masuda, K., Kurata, K. & Sakaguchi, M. (2007). Isolation and characterization of native Cry j 3 from Japanese cedar (Cryptomeria japonica) pollen. *Allergy*, Vol. 62, No. 5, pp. 547-553.

Futamura, N., Mukai, Y., Sakaguchi, M., Yasueda, H., Inouye, S., Midoro-Horiuti, T., Goldblum, R.M. & Shinohara, K. (2002). Isolation and characterization of cDNAs that encode homologs of a pathogenesis-related protein allergen from Cryptomeria japonica. *Bioscience, Biotechnology and Biochemistry*, Vol. 66, No. 11, pp. 2495-2500.

Futamura, N., Kusunoki, Y., Mukai, Y. & Shinohara, K. (2006). Characterization of genes for a pollen allergen, Cry j 2, of Cryptomeria japonica. *International Archives of Allergy and Immunology*, Vol. 28, No. 143 (1), pp. 59-68.

Gao, Z., E. W., Weg, E.W., Matos, C.I., Arens, P., Bolhaar, S.T.H.P., Knulst, A.C., Li, Y., Hoffmann-Sommergruber, K., & Gilissen, L.J.W.J. (2008). Assessment of allelic diversity in intron-containing Mal d 1 genes and their association to apple allergenicity. *BMC Plant Biology*, 8:116

Geller-Bernstein, C., Arad, G., Keynan, N., Lahoz, C., Cardaba, B. & Waisel, Y. (1996). Hypersensitivity to pollen of Olea europaea in Israel. *Allergy*, Vol. 51, No. 5, pp. 356-359.

Gilissen, L.J.W.J., Bolhaar, S.T.H.P., Knulst, A.C., Zuidmeer, L., van Ree, R., Gao, Z.S. & van de Weg, W.E. (2006a). Production of hypoallergenic plant foods by selection, breeding and genetic modification. In: Allergy matters. New approaches to allergy prevention and management. Gilissen, L.J.E.J., Wichers, H.J., Savelkoul, H.F.J. and Bogers, R.J. (Eds). *Wageningen UR Frontis Series*, Chapter 11, pp. 95-105.

Gilissen, L.J.W.J., Wichers, H.J., Savelkoul, H.F.J. & Beers, G. (2006b). Future developments in allergy prevention: a matter of integrating medical, natural and social sciences. In: Allergy matters. New approaches to allergy prevention and management. Gilissen,

L.J.E.J., Wichers, H.J., Savelkoul, H.F.J. and Bogers, R.J. (Eds). *Wageningen UR Frontis Series*, Chapter, 1, pp. 3-12.

Goto, Y., Kondo,T., Ide, T., Yasueda, H., Kuramoto, N. & Yamamoto, K. (2004). Cry j 1 isoforms derived from *Cryptomeria japonica* trees have different binding properties to monoclonal antibodies. *Clinical and Experimental Allergy*, Vol, 34, No. 11, pp. 1754-1761.

Goto-Fukuda, Y., Yasueda, H., Saito, A. & Kondo, T. (2007). Investigation of the variation of Cry j 2 concentration in pollen among sugi (*Cryptomeria japonica* d. Don) trees using a newly established extraction method. *Arerugi*, Vol. 56, No. 10, pp. 1262-1269.

Griffith, I.J., Lussier, A., Garman, R., Koury, R., Yeung, H. & Pollock, J. (1993). The cDNA cloning of Cry j 1, the major allergen of Cryptomeria japonica. *The Journal of Allergy and Clinical Immunology*, Vol. 91, p. 339.

Grote, M., Stumvoll, S., Reichelt, R., Lidholm, J. & Rudolf, V. (2002). Identification of an allergen related to Phl p 4, a major timothy grass pollen allergen, in pollens, vegetables, and fruits by immunogold electron microscopy. *Biological Chemistry*, Vol. 83, No. 9, pp. 1441-1445.

Grote, M., Vrtala, S. & Valenta, R. (1993). Monitoring of two allergens, Bet v I and profilin, in dry and rehydrated birch pollen by immunogold electron microscopy and immunoblotting.
The Journal of Histochemistry and Cytochemistry, Vol. 41, No. 5, pp. 745-750.

Hamman-Khalifa, A.M. (2005). Utilización de marcadores relacionados con la alergenicidad y la biosíntesis de lípidos para la discriminación entre cultivares de olivo. Doctoral thesis. Granada (Spain): University of Granada.

Hamman-Khalifa, A.M., Alché, J.D. & Rodríguez-García, M.I. (2003). Discriminación molecular en el polen de variedades españolas y marroquíes de olivo (*Olea europaea* L.). *Polen*. Vol. 13, pp. 219-225.

Hamman-Khalifa, A.M., Castro-López, A.J., Jiménez-López, J.C., Rodríguez-García, M.I., & Alché, J.D. (2008). Olive cultivar origin is a major cause of polymorphism for Ole e 1 pollen allergen. *BMC Plant Biology*, 8:10.

Hashimoto, M., Nigi, H., Sakaguchi, M., Inouye, S., Imaoka, K., Miyazawa, H., Taniguchi, Y., Kurimoto, M., Yasueda, H. & Ogawa, T. (1995). Sensitivity to two major allergens (Cry j I and Cry j II) in patients with Japanese Cedar (*Cryptomeria japonica*) pollinosis. *Clinical and Experimental Allergy*. Vol. 25, No. 9, pp. 848-852.

Helbling, A. (1997). Important cross-reactive allergens. *Schweiz Med Wochenschr*, Vol. 127, No. 10, pp. 382-389.

Hirschl, M.H. (1989). Isolation and characterization of birch pollen protein P13. *Wien Klin Wochenschr*, Vol. 101, No.19, pp. 679-681.

Holm, J., Baerentzen, G., Gajhede, M., Ipsen, H., Larsen, J.N., Lowenstein, H., Wissenbacha, M. & Spangforta, M.D. (2001). Molecular basis of allergic cross-reactivity between group 1 major allergens from birch and apple. *Journal of Chromatography B: Biomedical Sciences and Applications*, Vol. 756, No.1-2, pp. 307-313.

Hoppe, S., Neidhart, S., Zunker, K., Hutasingh, P., Carle, R., Steinhart, H. & Paschke, A. (2006). The influences of cultivar and thermal processing on the allergenic potency of lychees (*Litchi chinensis* SONN.). *Food Chemistry*, Vol. 96, No. 2, pp. 209-219.

Ibrahim, A.R., Kawamoto, S., Aki, T., Shimada, Y., Rikimaru, S., Onishi, N., Babiker, E.E., Oiso, I., Hashimoto, K., Hayashi, T. & Ono, K. (2010a). Molecular cloning and immunochemical characterization of a novel major japanese cedar pollen allergen belonging to the aspartic protease family. *International Archives of Allergy and Immunology*, Vol. 152, No. 3, pp. 207-218.

Ibrahim, A.R., Kawamoto, S., Mizuno, K., Shimada, Y., Rikimaru, S., Onishi, N., Hashimoto, K., Aki, T., Hayashi, T. & Ono, K. (2010b). Molecular cloning and immunochemical characterization of a new japanese cedar pollen allergen homologous to plant subtilisin-like serine protease. *World Allergy Organization Journal*, Vol. 3, No. 1, pp. 262-265.

Ibrahim, A.R., Kawamoto, S., Nishimura, M., Pak, S., Aki, T., Diaz-Perales, A., Salcedo, G., Asturias, J.A., Hayashi, T. & Ono, K. (2010c). A new lipid transfer protein homolog identified as an IgE-binding antigen from japanese cedar pollen. *Bioscience, Biotechnology, and Biochemistry*, Vol. 74, No. 3, pp. 504-509.

Ipsen, H., Bøwadt, H., Janniche, H., Nuchel Petersen, B., Munch, E.P., Wihl, J.A. & Løwenstein, H. (1985). Immunochemical characterization of reference alder (*Alnus glutinosa*) and hazel (*Corylus avellana*) pollen extracts and the partial immunochemical identity between the major allergens of alder, birch and hazel pollens. *Allergy*, Vol. 40, No. 7, pp.510-518.

Ito, H., Nishimura, J., Suzuki, M., Mamiya, S., Sato, K., Takagi, I. & Baba, S. (1995). Specific IgE to Japanese cypress (*Chamaecyparis obtusa*) in patients with nasal allergy. *Annals of Allergy, Asthma & Immunology*. Vol. 74, No. 4, pp. 299-303.

Jaradat, Z.W., Al Bzourb, A., Ababnehac, Q., Shdiefatd, S., Jaradatb, S. & Al Domie, H. (2012). Identification of allergenic pollen grains in 36 olive (Olea europaea) cultivars grown in Jordan. *Food and Agricultural Immunology*, Vol. 23, No. 3, pp. 255-264.

Jimenez-Lopez, J.C. (2008). Caracterización molecular del polimorfismo de las profilinas en el polen del olivo y otras especies alergogénicas. Doctoral thesis. Granada (Spain): University of Granada.

Jimenez-Lopez, J.C.; Kotchoni, S.O.; Rodríguez-García, M.I. & Alché, J.D. (2012a). Structure and functional features of olive pollen pectin methylesterase using homology modeling and molecular docking methods. *Journal of Molecular Modeling*. In press.

Jimenez-Lopez, J.C., Morales, S., Castro, A.J., Volkmann, D., Rodríguez-García, M.I. & Alché, J.D. (2012b). Characterization of profilin polymorphism in pollen with a focus on multifunctionality. *PLoS ONE*, Vol. 7, No. 2, e30878.

Jimenez-Lopez J.C., Rodríguez-García, M.I. & Alché J.D. (2011). Systematic and Phylogenetic Analysis of the Ole e 1 Pollen Protein Family Members in Plants. In: Systems and Computational Biology - Bioinformatics and Computational Modeling, Ning-Sun Yang (Ed.), *InTech*, pp. 245-260.

Jung, K., Schlenvoigt, G. & Jäger, L. (1987). Allergologic-immunochemical study of tree and bush pollen. III – Cross reactions of human IgE antibodies with various tree pollen allergens. *Allergie und Immunologie*, Vol. 33, No. 4, pp. 223-230.

Kang, I.H., Srivastava, P., Ozias-Akins, P. & Gallo, M. (2007). Temporal and spatial expression of the major allergens in developing and germinating peanut seed. *Plant Physiology*, Vol. 144, No. 2, pp. 836-45.

Karamloo, F., Schmitz, N., Scheurer, S., Foetisch, K., Hoffman, A., Haustein, D. & Vieths, S. (1999). Molecular cloning and characterization of a birch pollen minor allergen, Bet v 5, belonging to a family of isoflavone reductase-related proteins. *The Journal of Allergy and Clinical Immunology*, Vol. 104, No. 5, pp. 991-999 .

Karamloo, F., Wangorsch, A., Kasahara, H., Davin, L.B., Haustein, D., Lewis, N.G. & Vieths, S.
(2001). Phenylcoumaran benzylic ether and isoflavonoid reductases are a new class of cross-reactive allergens in birch pollen, fruits and vegetables. *European Journal of Biochemistry*, Vol. 268, No. 20, pp. 5310-5320.

Kawamoto, S., Fujimura, T., Nishida, M., Tanaka, T., Aki, T., Masubuchi, M., Hayashi, T., Suzuki, O., Shigeta, S. & Ono, K. (2002). Molecular cloning and characterization of a new Japanese cedar pollen allergen homologous to plant isoflavone reductase family. *Clinical and Experimental Allergy*, Vol. 32, No. 7, pp. 1064-1070.

Khadari, B., Breton, C., Moutier, N., Roger, J.P., Besnard, G., Bervillé, A. & Dosba, F. (2003). The use of molecular markers for germplasm management in a French olive collection. *Theoretical and Applied Genetics*, Vol. 106, No. 3, pp. 521-529.

Kimura, Y., Kuroki, M., Maeda, M., Okano, M., Yokoyama, M. & Kino, K. (2008). Glycoform analysis of Japanese cypress pollen allergen, Cha o 1: a comparison of the glycoforms of cedar and cypress pollen allergens. *Bioscience, Biotechnology, and Biochemistry*, Vol. 72, No. 2, pp. 485-491.

Komiyama, N., Sone, T., Shimizu, K., Morikubo, K. & Kino, K. (1994). cDNA cloning and expression of Cry j II the second major allergen of Japanese cedar pollen. *Biochemical and Biophysical Research Communications*, Vol. 201, No. 2, pp. 1021-1028.

Kondo, Y., Ipsen, H., Lowenstein, H., Karpas, A. & Hsieh, L.S. (1997). Comparison of concentrations of Cry j 1 and Cry j 2 in diploid and triploid Japanese Cedar (*Cryptomeria japonica*) pollen extracts. *Allergy*, Vol. 52, No. 4, pp. 455-459.

Kondo, Y., Tokuda, R., Urisu, A. & Matsuda, T. (2002). Assessment of cross-reactivity between Japanese cedar (*Cryptomeria japonica*) pollen and tomato fruit extracts by RAST inhibition and immunoblot inhibition. *Clinical and Experimental Allergy, Vol. 32, No. 4, pp. 590-594.*

Kos, T., Hoffmann-Sommergruber, K., Ferreira, F., Hirschwehr, R., Ahorn, H., Horak, F., Jäger, S., Sperr, W., Kraft, D. & Scheiner, O. (1993). Purification, characterization and N-terminal amino acid sequence of a new major allergen from European chestnut pollen – Cas s 1. *Biochemical and Biophysical Research Communications*, Vol. 196, No. 3, pp. 1086-1092.

Kottapallia, K.R., Paytonb, P., Rakwalc, R., Agrawald, G. K., Shibatoc, J., Burowa, M. & Puppalaf, N. (2008). Proteomics analysis of mature seed of four peanut cultivars using two-dimensional gel electrophoresis reveals distinct differential expression of storage, anti-nutritional, and allergenic proteins. *Plant Science*, Vol. 175, No. 3, pp. 321–329.

Kwaasi, A.A., Harfi, H.A., Parhar, R.S., Al-Sedairy, S.T., Collison, K.S., Panzani, R.C. & Al-Mohanna, F.A. (1999). Allergy to Date fruits: characterization of antigens and allergens of fruits of the Date Palm (*Phoenix dactylifera* L.). *Allergy*, Vol. 54, No. 12, pp. 1270-1277.

Kwaasi, A.A., Harfi, H.A., Parhar, R.S., Collison, K.S., Al-Sedairy, S.T. & Al-Mohanna, F.A. (2000). Cultivar-specific IgE-epitopes in Date (*Phoenix dactylifera* L.) fruit allergy. Correlation of skin test reactivity and IgE-binding properties in selecting Date cultivars for allergen standardization. *International Archives of Allergy and Immunology,* Vol. 123, No. 2, pp. 137-144.

Kwaasi, A.A., Parhar, R.S., Tipirneni, P., Harfi, H.A. & al-Sedairy, S.T. (1994). Cultivar-specific epitopes in date palm (*Phoenix dactylifera* L.) pollenosis. Differential antigenic and allergenic properties of pollen from ten cultivars. *International Archives of Allergy and Immunology,* Vol. 104, No. 3, pp. 281-90.

La Mantia, M., Lain, O., Caruso, T. & Testolin, R. (2005). SSR-based DNA fingerprints reveal the genetic diversity of Sicilian olive (*Olea europaea* L.) germplasm. *The journal of Horticultural Science & Biotechnology,* Vol. 80, No. 8, pp. 628-632.

Lacovacci, P., Afferni, C., Butteroni, C., Pironi, L., Puggioni, E.M., Orlandi, A., Barletta, B., Tinghino, R., Ariano, R., Panzani, R.C., Di Felice, G. & Pini, C. (2002). Comparison between the native glycosylated and the recombinant Cup a1 allergen: role of carbohydrates in the histamine release from basophils. *Clinical and Experimental Allergy,* Vol. 32, No.11, pp. 1620-1627.

Leduc, V., Charpin, D., Aparicio, C., Veber, C. & Guerin, L. (2000). Allergy to cypress pollen: preparation of a reference and standardization extract in vivo. *Allergie et Immunologie,* Vol. 32, No. 3, pp. 101-103.

Maeda, M., Kamamoto, M., Hino, K., Yamamoto, S., Kimura, M., Okano, M. & Kimura, Y. (2005). Glycoform analysis of Japanese cedar pollen allergen, Cry j 1. *Bioscience, Biotechnology, and Biochemistry,* Vol. 69, No.9, pp. 1700-1705.

Mari, A., Rasi, C., Palazzo, P. & Scala, E. (2009). Allergen databases: current status and perspectives. *Current Allergy and Asthma Reports,* Vol. 9, pp. 376-83.

Maruyama-Funstsuki, W., Fujino, K., Suzuki, T. & Funatsuki, H. (2004). Quantification of a major allergenic protein in common buckwheat cultivars by an enzyme-linked immunosorbent assay (ELISA). *Fagopyrum,* Vol, 21, pp. 39-44.

Matsumura, D., Nabe, T., Mizutani, N., Fujii, M. & Kohno, S. (2006). Detection of new antigenic proteins in Japanese cedar pollen. *Biological & pharmaceutical bulletin,* Vol. 29, No. 6, pp. 1162-1166.

Matthes, A. & Schmitz-Eiberger, M. (2009). Apple (*Malus domestica* L. Borkh.) allergen Mal d 1: effect of cultivar, cultivation system, and storage conditions. *Journal of Agricultural and Food Chemistry,* Vol. 57, No. 22, pp. 10548-10553.

McNeill, J., Barrie, F.R., Burdet, H.M., Demoulin, V., Hawksworth, D.L., Marhold, K., Nocolson, D.H., Prado, J., Silva, P.C., Skog, J.E., Wiersema, J.H. & Turland, N.J. (2006). International Code of Botanical Nomenclature (Vienna Code). *Regnum Vegetabile 146. A.R.G. Gantner Verlag KG.*

Midoro-Horiuti, T., Goldblum, R.M., Kurosky, A., Goetz, D.W. & Brooks, E.G. (1999). Isolation and characterization of the mountain Cedar (*Juniperus ashei*) pollen major allergen, Jun a 1. *The Journal of Allergy and Clinical Immunology,* Vol. 104, No. 3 (Pt 1), pp. 608-612.

Midoro-Horiuti, T., Schein, C.H., Mathura, V., Braun, W., Czerwinski, E.W., Togawa, A., Kondo, Y., Oka, T., Watanabe, M. & Goldblum, R.M. (2006). Structural basis for epitope sharing between group 1 allergens of cedar pollen. *Molecular Immunology*, Vol. 43, No.6, pp. 509-518.

Mistrello, G., Roncarolo, D., Zanoni, D., Zanotta, S., Amato, S., Falagiani, P. & Ariano, R. (2002). Allergenic relevance of *Cupressus arizonica* pollen extract and biological characterization of the allergoid. *International Archives of Allergy and Immunology*, Vol. 129, No. 4, pp. 296-304.

Mogensen, J.E., Wimmer, R., Larsen, J.N., Spangfort, M.D. & Otzen, D.E. (2002). The major birch allergen, Bet v 1, shows affinity for a broad spectrum of physiological ligands. *The Journal of Biological Chemistry*, Vol. 277, No. 26, pp. 23684-23692.

Mohapatra, S.S., Lockey, R.F., & Polo, F. (2004). Weed pollen allergens. Allergens and Allergen Immunotherapy. Marcel Dekker, Inc. New York, pp. 207-222.

Morales, S. (2012). Desarrollo y aplicación de un sistema multiplex para la caracterización del polimorfismo de las proteínas alergénicas en el polen de distintas variedades de olivo (*Olea europaea* L.). Doctoral thesis. Granada (Spain): University of Granada.

Morales, S., Castro, A.J., Jiménez-López, J.C., Florido, F., Rodríguez-García, M.I. & Alché, J.D. (2012). A novel multiplex method for the simultaneous detection and relative quantification of pollen allergens. *Electrophoresis*, Vol. 33, No. 9-10, pp.1367-1374.

Morales, S., Jiménez-López, J.C., Castro, A.J., Rodríguez-García, M.I. & Alché, J.D. (2008). Olive pollen profilin (Ole e 2 allergen) co-localizes with highly active areas of the actin cytoskeleton and is released to the culture medium during in vitro pollen germination. *Journal of Microscopy-Oxford*, Vol. 231, No. 2, pp. 332-342.

Moreno-Aguilar, C. (2008). Improving pollen immunotherapy: minor allergens and panallergens. *Allergologia et Immunopathologia*, Vol. 36, No. 1, pp. 26:30.

Mothes, N., Horak, F. & Valenta, R. (2004). Transition from a botanical to a molecular classification in tree pollen allergy: implications for diagnosis and therapy. *International Archives of Allergy and Immunology*, Vol. 135, No. 4, pp. 357-373.

Mothes, N., Westritschnig, K. & Valenta, R. (2004). Tree pollen allergens. *Clinical Allergy and Immunology*, Vol. 18, pp. 165-84.

Moverare, R., Westritschnig, K., Svensson, M., Hayek, B., Bende, M., Pauli, G., Sorva, R., Haahtela, T., Valenta, R. & Elfman, L. (2002). Different IgE Reactivity Profiles in Birch Pollen-Sensitive Patients from Six European Populations Revealed by Recombinant Allergens: An Imprint of Local Sensitization. *International Archives of Allergy and Immunology*, Vol. 128, No. 4, pp. 325-335.

Muñoz, C., Hoffmann, T., Medina Escobar, N., Ludemann, F., Botella, M.A., Valpuesta, V. & Schwab, W. (2010). The strawberry fruit Fra a allergen functions in flavonoid biosynthesis. *Molecular Plant*, Vol. 3, No. 1, pp. 113-124.

Muzzalupo, I.; Lombardo, N.; Musacchio, A.; Noce, M.E.; Pellegrino, G.; Perri, E. & Sajjad, A. (2006). DNA sequence analysis of microsatellite markers enhances their efficiency for germplasm management in an Italian olive collection. *Journal of the American Society for Horticultural Science*, Vol. 131, pp. 352-359.

Nair, A. & Adachi, T. (2002). Screening and selection of hypoallergenic buckwheat species. *The Scientific World Journal*, Vol. 2, pp. 818–826.

Nakamura, A., Tanabe, S., Watanabe, J. & Makino, T. (2005). Primary screening of relatively less allergenic wheat varieties. *Journal of Nutritional Science and Vitaminology*, Vol. 51, No. 13, pp. 204-206.

Namba, M., Kurose, M., Torigoe, K., Hino, K., Taniguchi, Y., Fukuda, S., Usui, M. & Kurimoto, M. (1994). Molecular cloning of the second major allergen, Cry j II, from Japanese cedar pollen. *FEBS Letters*, No. 353(2), pp. 124-128.

Napoli, A., Aiello, D., Di Donna, L., Moschidis, P. & Sindona, G. (2008). Vegetable Proteomics: The Detection of Ole e 1 Isoallergens by Peptide Matching of MALDI MS/MS Spectra of Underivatized and Dansylated Glycopeptides. *Journal of Proteome Research*, Vol. 7, No. 7, pp 2723–2732.

Napoli, A., Aiello, D., Di Donna, L., Sajjad, A., Perri, E. & Sindona, G. (2006). Profiling of hydrophilic proteins from *Olea europaea* olive pollen by MALDI TOF mass spectrometry. *Analytical Chemistry*, Vol 78, No. 10, pp. 3434-3443.

Niederberger, V., Laffer, S., Froschl, R., Kraft, D., Rumpold, H., Kapiotis, S., Valenta, R. & Spitzauer, S. (1998). IgE antibodies to recombinant pollen allergens (Phl p 1, Phl p 2, Phl p 5, and Bet v 2) account for a high percentage of grass pollen-specific IgE. *The Journal of Allergy and Clinical Immunology*, Vol. 101, No. 2 (Pt 1), pp. 258-264.

Ohtsuki, T., Taniguchi, Y., Kohno, K., Fukuda, S., Usui, M. & Kurimoto, M. (1995). Cry j 2, a major allergen of Japanese cedar pollen, shows polymethylgalacturonase activity. *Allergy*, Vol. 50, No. 6, pp. 483-488.

Okano, M., Kimura, Y., Kino, K., Michigami, Y., Sakamoto, S., Sugata, Y., Maeda, M., Matsuda, F., Kimura, M., Ogawa, T. & Nishizaki, K. (2004). Roles of major oligosaccharides on Cry j 1 in human immunoglobulin E and T cell responses. *Clinical and Experimental Allergy*, Vol. 34, No. 5, pp.770-778.

Okano, M., Kino, K., Takishita, T., Hattori, H., Ogawa, T., Yoshino, T., Yokoyama, M. & Nishizaki, K. (2001). Roles of carbohydrates on Cry j 1, the major allergen of Japanese cedar pollen, in specific T-cell responses. *The Journal of Allergy and Clinical Immunology*, Vol. 108, No. 1, pp. 101-108.

Ouazzani, N., Lumaret, R., Villemur, P. & Di Giusto, F. (1993). Leaf allozyme variation in cultivated and wild Olive trees (*Olea europaea* L.). *Journal of Heredity*, Vol. 84, No.1, pp. 34-42.

Panzani, R., Yasueda, H., Shimizu, T. & Shida, T. (1986). Cross-reactivity between the pollens of *Cupressus sempervirens* (common cypress) and of *Cryptomeria japonica* (Japanese Cedar). *Annals of Allergy*, Vol. 57, No. 1, pp. 26-30.

Pauli, G., Bessot, J.C., Dietemann-Molard, A., Braun, P.A. & Thierry, R. (1985). Celery sensitivity: clinical and immunological correlations with pollen allergy. *Clinical Allergy*, Vol. 15, No. 3, pp. 273-279.

Penon, J.P. (2000). Cypress arizona: allergic extracts with a diagnostic purpose. *Allergie et Immunologie*, Vol. 32, No. 3, pp. 107-108.

Pharmacia Diagnostics AB (2001). Allergenic Plants. Systematics of common and rare allergens. Version 2.0 CD.

Postigo, I., Guisantes, J.A., Negro, J.M., Rodriguez-Pacheco, R., David-Garcia, D. & Martinez, J. (2009). Identification of 2 new allergens of *Phoenix dactylifera* using an immunoproteomics approach. *Journal of Investigational Allergology & Clinical Immunology*, Vol. 19, No. 6, pp. 504-507.

Radauer, C. & Breiteneder, H. (2006). Pollen allergens are restricted to few protein families and show distinct patterns of species distribution. *Journal of Allergy and Clinical Immunology*, Vol. 117, No. 1, pp. 141–147.

Ribeiro, H., Cunha, M., Calado, L. & Abreu, I. (2012). Pollen morphology and quality of twenty olive (*Olea europaea* L.) cultivars grown in Portugal. *Acta Horticulturae (ISHS)*, Vol. 949, pp. 259-

Rur, Mira. (2007). Localization of the main allergy protein in two apple cultivars grown in Sweden. *Bachelor project in the Danish-Swedish Horticulture programme*, Vol. 2007, No.3, 23 pages.

Saito, M. & Teranishi, H. (2002). Immunologic determination of the major allergen, Cry j 1, in *Cryptomeria japonica* pollen of 117 clones in Toyama prefecture: Some implications for further forestry research in pollinosis prevention. *Allergology International*, Vol. 51, No. 3, pp. 191–195.

Sakaguchi, M., Inouye, S., Taniai, M., Ando, S., Usui, M. & Matuhasi, T. (1990). Identification of the second major allergen of Japanese Cedar pollen. *Allergy*, Vol. 45, No. 4, pp. 309-312.

Scheiner, O. (1993). Molecular and functional characterization of allergens: fundamental and practical aspects. *Wien Klin Wochenschr*, Vol. 105, No. 22, pp. 653-658.

Schenk, M.F., Cordewener , J.H.G., America, A.H.P., Peters, J., Smulders, M.J.M. & Gilissen, L.J.W.J. (2011). Proteomic analysis of the major birch allergen Bet v 1 predicts allergenicity for 15 birch species. *Journal of Proteomics*, Vol. 74, No. 8, pp. 1290–1300.

Schenk, M.F., Cordewener , J.H.G., America, A.H.P., Peters, J., van't Westende W.P.C., Smulders, M.J.M. & Gilissen, L.J.W.J. (2009). Characterization of PR-10 genes from eight Betula species and detection of Bet v 1 isoforms in birch pollen. *BMC Plant Biology* 9:24

Schenk, M.F., Gilissen, L.J.W.J., Esselink, G.D. & Smulders, M.J.M. (2006). Seven different genes encode a diverse mixture of isoforms of Bet v 1, the major birch pollen allergen. *BMC Genomics*, Vol. 7, p. 168.

Schenk, M.F., Thienpont, C.N., Koopman, W.J. M., Gilissen, L.J. W. J. & Smulders, M.J. M. (2008). Phylogenetic relationships in Betula (Betulaceae) based on AFLP markers. *Tree Genetics & Genomes*, Vol. 4, No. 4, pp. 911-924.

Seiberler, S., Scheiner, O., Kraft, D., Lonsdale, D. & Valenta, R. (1994). Characterization of a birch pollen allergen, Bet v III, representing a novel class of Ca^{2+} binding proteins: specific expression in mature pollen and dependence of patient's IgE binding on protein-bound Ca^{2+}. *The EMBO Journal*, Vol. 13, No. 15, pp. 3481-3486.

Shahali, Y., Majd, A., Pourpak, Z., Tajadod, G., Haftlang, M. & Moin, M. (2007). Comparative study of the pollen protein contents in two major varieties of *Cupressus arizonica* planted in Tehran. *Iranian Journal of Allergy, Asthma and Immunology*, Vol. 6 No. 3, pp.123-127.

Skamstrup-Hansen, K., Vieths, S., Vestergaard, H., Stahl Skov, P., Bindslev-Jensen, C. & Poulsen, L.K. (2001). Seasonal variation in food allergy to apple. *Journal of Chromatography,* Vol. 756, No. 1-2, pp. 19– 32.

Soleimani, A., Alché, J.D., Castro, A.J., Rodríguez-García, M.I. & Ladan Moghadam, A.R. (2012). Using Two-Dimensional Gel Electrophoresis approach for characterizing of the Ole e 1, an olive pollen major allergen. *Acta Horticulturae (ISHS),* Vol. 932, pp. 69-72.

Soleimani, A., Morales, S., Jiménez-López, J.C., Castro A.J., Rodríguez-García, M.I. & Alché, J.D. (2012). Differential expression and sequence polymorphism of the olive pollen allergen Ole e 1 in two Iranian cultivars. *Iranian Journal of Allergy, Asthma and Immunology,* in press.

Sone, T., Komiyama, N., Shimizu, K., Kusakabe, T., Morikubo, K. & Kino, K. (1994). Cloning and sequencing of cDNA coding for Cry j I, a major allergen of Japanese cedar pollen. *Biochemical and Biophysical Research Communications,* Vol. 199, No. 2, pp. 619-625.

Spangenberg,G., Petrovska, N., Kearney, G.A. & Smith, K.F.(2006). Low-pollen-allergen ryegrasses: towards a continent free of hay fever? In: Allergy Matters: New approaches to allergy prevention and management. *Wageningen UR Frontis Series.* Chapter 13, pp. 121-128.

Stäger, J., Wüthrich, B. & Johansson, S.G.O. (1991). Spice allergy in celery-sensitive patients. *Allergy, Vol.* 46, No. 6, pp. 475-478.

Stewart, G.A. & McWilliam, A.S. (2001). Endogenous function and biological significance of aeroallergens: an update. *Current Opinion in Allergy and Clinical Immunology,* Vol. 1, No. 1, pp. 95-103.

Suárez-Cervera, M., Castells, T., Vega-Maray, A., Civantos, E., del Pozo, V., Fernandez-Gonzalez, D., Moreno-Grau, S., Moral, A., Lopez-Iglesias, C., Lahoz, C. & Seoane-Camba, J.A. (2008). Effects of air pollution on Cup a 3 allergen in *Cupressus arizonica* pollen grains. A*nnals of Allergy, Asthma & Immunology,* Vol. 101, No. 1, pp. 57-66.

Susani, M., Jertschin, P., Dolecek, C., Sperr, W.R., Valent, P., Ebner, C., Kraft, D., Valenta, R. & Scheiner, O. (1995). High level expression of birch pollen profilin (Bet v 2) in *Escherichia coli*: purification and characterization of the recombinant allergen. *Biochemical and Biophysical Research Communications,* Vol. 215, No. 1, pp. 250-263.

Swoboda, I., Scheiner, O., Kraft, D., Breitenbach, M., Heberle-Bors, E. & Vicente, O. (1994). A birch gene family encoding pollen allergens and pathogenesis-related proteins. *Biochimica et Biophysica Acta,* Vol. 1219, No. 2, pp. 457-464.

Takahashi, Y. & Aoyama, M. (2006). Development of the simple method for measurement the content of Cry j 1 in the air by latex agglutination test. *Arerugi,* Vol. 55, No. 1, pp. 28-33.

Takhtajan, A. (1997). Diversity and classification of flowering plants. *Columbia University Press, New York,* 643 pages.

Taneichi, M., Uehara, M. & Katagiri, M. (1994). Analysis of birch pollen allergen. *Hokkaido Igaku Zasshi,* Vol. 69, No. 5, pp. 1154-1161.

Taniai, M., Ando, S., Usui, M., Kurimoto, M., Sakaguchi, M., Inouye, S. & Matuhasi, T. (1988). N-terminal amino acid sequence of a major allergen of Japanese cedar pollen (Cry j 1). *FEBS Letters,* Vol. 239, No. 2, pp. 329-332.

Taniguchi, Y., Ono, A., Sawatani, M., Nanba, M., Kohno, K., Usui, M., Kurimoto, M. & Matuhasi, T. (1995). Cry j 1, a major allergen of Japanese cedar pollen, has pectate lyase enzyme activity. *Allergy*, Vol. 50, No. 1, pp. 90-93.

Tinghino, R., Twardosz, A., Barletta, B., Puggioni, E.M., Iacovacci, P., Butteroni, C., Afferni, C., Mari, A., Hayek, B., Di Felice, G., Focke, M., Westritschnig, K., Valenta, R. & Pini, C. (2002). Molecular, structural, and immunologic relationships between different families of recombinant calcium-binding pollen allergens. *The Journal of Allergy and Clinical Immunology*, Vol. 109, No.2 (Pt 1), pp. 314-320.

Togawa, A., Panzani, R.C., Garza, M.A., Kishikawa, R., Goldblum, R.M. & Midoro-Horiuti, T. (2006). Identification of italian cypress (*Cupressus sempervirens*) pollen allergen Cup s 3 using homology and cross-reactivity. *Annals of Allergy, Asthma & Immunology*, Vol. 97 No. 3, pp. 336-342.

Trujillo I. & Rallo, L. (1995). Identifying olive cultivars by isozyme analysis. *Journal of the American Society for Horticultural Science*, Vol. 120, pp. 318-324.

Twardosz, A., Hayek, B., Seiberler, S., Vangelista, L., Elfman, L., Grönlund, H., Kraft, D. & Valenta, R. (1997). Molecular characterization, expression in Escherichia coli, and epitope analysis of a two EF-hand calcium-binding birch pollen allergen, Bet v 4. *Biochemical and Biophysics Research Communications*, Vol. 239, No. 1, pp. 197-204.

Valenta, R., Breiteneder, H., Petternburger, K., Breitenbach, M., Rumpold, H., Kraft, D. & Scheiner, O. (1991a). Homology of the major birch-pollen allergen, Bet v I, with the major pollen allergens of alder, hazel, and hornbeam at the nucleic acid level as determined by cross-hybridization. *The Journal of Allergy and Clinical Immunology*, Vol. 87, No. 3, pp. 677-682.

Valenta, R., Duchêne, M., Breitenbach, M., Pettenburger, K., Koller, L., Rumpold, H., Scheiner, O. & Kraft, D. (1991b). A low molecular weight allergen of white birch (*Betula verrucosa*) is highly homologous to human profilin. *International Archives of Allergy and Applied Immunology*, Vol, 94, No. 1-4, pp. 368-370.

Valenta, R., Duchêne, M., Pettenburger, K., Sillaber, C., Valent, P., Bettelheim, P., Breitenbach, M., Rumpold, H., Kraft, D. & Scheiner, O. (1991c). Identification of profilin as a novel pollen allergen; IgE autoreactivity in sensitised individuals. *Science*, Vol. 253, No. 5019, pp. 557-560.

Valenta, R., Ferreira, F., Grote, M., Swoboda, I., Vrtala, S., Duchêne, M., Deviller, P., Meagher, R.B., McKinney, E., Heberle-Bors, E., Krafts, D. & Scheiners, O. (1993). Identification of profilin as an actin-binding protein in higher plants. *The Journal of Biological Chemistry*, Vol. 268, No. 30, pp. 22777-22781.

Van Ree, R. (2002). Isoallergens: a clinically relevant phenomenon or just a product of cloning?. *Clinical and Experimental Allergy*. Vol. 32, pp. 975-978.

Vieths, S., Frank, E., Scheurer, S., Meyer, H.E., Hrazdina, G. & Haustein, D. (1998). Characterization of a new IgE-binding 35-kDa protein from birch pollen with cross-reacting homologues in various plant foods. *Scandinavian Journal of Immunology*, Vol. 47, No. 3, pp. 263-272.

Vieths, S., Jankiewicz, A., Schöning, B. & Aulepp, H. (1994). Apple allergy: the IgE-binding potency of apple strains is related to the occurence of the 18-kDa allergen. *Allergy, Vol.* 49, No. 4, pp. 262– 271.

Vieths, S., Scheurer, S. & Ballmer-Weber, B. (2002). Current understanding of cross-reactivity of food allergens and pollen. *Annals of the New York Academy of Sciences,* Vol. 964, pp. 47-68.

Vlieg-Boerstra, B.J., van de Weg, W.E., van der Heide, S., Kerkhof, M., Arens, P., Heijerman-Peppelman, G. & Dubois, A. E. (2011). Identification of low allergenic apple cultivars using skin prick tests and oral food challenges. *Allergy,* Vol. 66, No. 4, pp. 491–498.

Wahl, R., Schmid Grendelmeier, P., Cromwell, O. & Wüthrich, B. (1996). *In vitro* investigation of cross-reactivity between birch and ash pollen allergen extracts. *The Journal of Allergy and Clinical Immunology,* Vol. 98, No. 1, pp. 99-106.

Waisel, Y. & Geller-Bernstein, C. (1996). Reliability of olive pollen extracts for skin prick tests. *Journal of Allergy and Clinical Immunology,* Vol. 98, No. 3, pp. 715-716.

Wallner, M., Erler, A., Hauser, M., Klinglmayr, E., Gardemaier, G., Vogel, L., Mari, A., Bohle, B., Briza, P. & Ferreira, F. (2009a). Immunologic characterization of isoforms of Car b 1 and Que a 1, the major hornbeam and oak pollen allergens. *Allergy,* Vol. 64, No. 3, pp. 452-460.

Wallner, M., Himly, M., Neubauer, A., Erler, A., Hauser, M., Asam, C., Mutschlechner, S., Ebner, C., Briza, P. & Ferreira, F. (2009b). The influence of recombinant production on the immunologic behavior of birch pollen isoallergens. *PLoS ONE,* Vol. 4, No. 12: e8457.

Wiebicke, K., Schlenvoigt, G. & Jäger, L. (1987). Allergologic-immunochemical study of various tree pollens. I. Characterization of antigen and allergen components in birch, beech, alder, hazel and oak pollens. *Allergie und Immunologie,* Vol. 33, No. 3, pp. 181-190.

Wiedemann, P., Giehl, K., Almo, S.C., Fedorov, A.A., Girvin, M., Steinberger, P., Rudiger, M., Ortner, M., Sippl, M., Dolecek, C., Kraft, D., Jockusch, B. & Valenta, R. (1996). Molecular and structural analysis of a continuous birch profilin epitope defined by a monoclonal antibody. *The Journal of Biological Chemistry,* Vol. 271, No. 47, pp. 29915-29921.

Wüthrich, B. & Dietschi, R. (1985). The celery-carrot-mugwort-condiment syndrome: skin test and RAST results. *Schweiz Med Wochenschr,* Vol. 115, No. 11, pp. 258-264.

Yasueda, H., Yui, Y., Shimizu, T. & Shida, T. (1983). Isolation and partial characterization of the major allergen from Japanese cedar (*Cryptomeria japonica*) pollen. *The Journal of Allergy and Clinical Immunology,* Vol. 71, No. 1 (Pt 1), pp. 77-86.

Yman L. (1982). Botanical relations and immunological cross-reactions in pollen allergy. *2nd ed. Pharmacia Diagnostics AB*. Uppsala. Sweden.

Yman L. (2001). Allergenic Plants. Systematics of common and rare allergens. *Version 2.0. CD-ROM. Pharmacia Diagnostics*. Uppsala, Sweden.

Zafra, A. (2007). Caracterización preliminar del polimorfismo de la proteína alergénica Ole e 5 en el polen del olivo de distintos cultivares. Master thesis. Granada (Spain): University of Granada.

Chapter 2

Clustering of Olive Pollens into Model Cultivars on the Basis of Their Allergenic Content

Sonia Morales, Antonio Jesús Castro,
Carmen Salmerón, Francisco Manuel Marco,
María Isabel Rodríguez-García and Juan de Dios Alché

Additional information is available at the end of the chapter

http://dx.doi.org/10.5772/49964

1. Introduction

Olive pollen allergy is a leading cause of seasonal allergic disease in the Mediterranean countries, where olive trees are intensively cultivated and pollen grain count reaches very high levels during the pollination season (Wheeler, 1992, Liccardi et al., 1996). The level of sensitization to olive pollen among the general population is directly related to the abundance of trees as this determines allergen exposure. Nevertheless, apart from tree abundance, other factors such as genetic background may influence the incidence of sensitization to olive pollen even in areas of very high exposition (Geller-Bernstein et al. 1996).Olive trees have been cultivated in the Mediterranean basin for several millennia and this has led to the selection of a wide variety of cultivars with agronomic importance. Olive germplasm is exceptionally wide, with more than 250 cultivars only in Spain (Barranco and Rallo, 2005), probably as a direct consequence of intensive cultivation.

Material commonly used for clinical and biological analysis corresponds in most cases to commercially available pollen, obtained from uncertain varietal sources. Previous studies have determined that most allergens isolated and characterized up to date are highly polymorphic (Villalba et al. 1993, 1994; Lombardero et al. 1994; Asturias et al. 1997; Alché et al. 1998; Tejera et al. 1999; Huecas et al. 2001; Martínez et al. 2002; Jiménez-López et al. 2012). Besides polymorphism, olive cultivars display broad differences in the expression levels for many allergens (Carnés et al. 2002; Conde Hernandez et al. 2002; Castro et al. 2003; Morales 2012) as well as in the number and molecular characteristics of the expressed allergen isoforms (Hamman-Khalifa et al. 2003, 2008; Hamman-Khalifa 2005; Castro et al. 2010; Jiménez-López et al. 2012). These differences are in a certain degree maintained over the years, and have been demonstrated to be associated to the genetic background of the different olive cultivars (Fernandez Caldas et al. 2007; Morales 2012; Morales et al. this volume). Differences in the allergen composition of the extracts, particularly as regard to the olive pollen major allergen Ole e 1, are responsible of large differences in the biological potency of the extracts. Thus, Castro et al. (2003) analysed the allergenicity and Ole e 1 content in pollen samples of 10 cultivars of olive trees, and compared it to a commercial extract with no indication on varietal origin, probably representing a mixture of several cultivars. The authors found that there are important differences in the content of this major allergen and that Ole e 1 abundance correlated with total allergenicity when extracts were tested by skin prick test (SPT) on allergic patients. Interestingly some patients (about 10%) did not react with a commercial extract and only reacted to extracts coming from specific cultivars. These findings may have important implications in both diagnosis and therapy of olive pollen allergy, and in the efficacy and safety of the preparations used for specific immunotherapy (SIT) (Castro et al., 2003; Alché et al. 2007; Hamman-Khalifa et al. 2008; Jiménez-López 2008; Morales 2012).

The basis for personalized SIT, based in the individual usage of olive cultivar extracts, have been described and are protected by several Spanish patents (Alché et al. 2005, 2006). However, and as handling and characterization of a large number of cultivar extracts is impracticable under industrial and clinical standards, the present work intends to define a limited number of model cultivar, characterized by distinctive pollen allergen profiles. For this purpose, a number of olive pollen extracts have been analysed in their content for several relevant allergens. After appropriate quantitation, several model cultivars have been defined to group the cultivars analysed. This model can be used as the basis for a future classification and inclusion of the numerous olive cultivars available.

2. Materials and methods

2.1. Pollen samples

Olea europaea L. pollen samples were obtained during May and June of 2005-2010 from cultivated trees of the following cultivars: 'Picual', 'Manzanilla', 'Arbequina', 'Blanqueta', 'Cornicabra', 'Verdial', 'Lechín', 'Hojiblanca', 'Lucio'and 'Loaime'. Pollen samples were collected from numerous branches of at least two trees of each cultivar by shaking flowering shoots inside paper bags. Prior to its storage in liquid nitrogen, the harvested pollen was sieved through a 150 μm mesh in order to eliminate fallen corollas, anthers and other rests. After light microscopy observation, foreign-species pollen was estimated to be <0.1% and other plant parts <0.5% for all the cultivars used.

2.2. Preparation of crude protein extracts and SDS-PAGE

Crude protein extracts were obtained by stirring 1 g of pollen for each cultivar in 10 ml extraction buffer (0.01 M ammonium bicarbonate, pH 8.0, and 2 mM phenylmethylsulfonyl fluoride) for 8 h at 4°C. After centrifugation (2 x 30 minutes at 14,000 rpm at 4°C), the supernatants were filtered through a 0.2 μm filter, and stored in aliquots at –20°C. Protein concentration in the different samples was measured using the Bio-Rad reagent (Bio-Rad, Hercules, CA, USA) and bovine serum albumin (BSA) as standard.

Proteins (30 μg per lane) and Mw1 (New England BioLabs, Ipswich, MA, USA) and Mw2 standards (MBI Fermentas, Vilnius, Lithuania) were separated by sodium dodecyl sulfate-polyacrylamide gel electrophoresis (SDS-PAGE) in 15% gels in a MiniProtean II system (Bio-Rad). The resulting gels were stained with Coomassie blue. The same procedure described here was applied to a commercially available extract used for olive pollen allergy diagnosis.

2.3. Immunoblotting

Gels obtained as described above were transferred onto BioTrace® polyvinylidene difluoride (PVDF) membranes (Pall BioSupport, Port Washington, NY, USA) at 100 V for 1.5 hours using a Mini Trans-Blot Electrophoretic Transfer Cell (Bio-Rad). Immunoblots were performed independently in the case of Ole e 1 (Figure 2) and Ole e 2 (Figure 3). Ole e 5 and Ole e 9 were simultaneously detected in the same membrane (Figure 4). Prior to the treatment with antibodies, the membranes were blocked with TBST buffer (Tris buffered saline: TBS + 0.3% v/v Tween 20) + 10% w/v dried skimmed milk.

The membranes were probed with antibodies to the following allergenic proteins: Ole e 1, (olive pollen major allergen), Ole e 2 (profilin), Ole e 5 (Cu,Zn superoxide dismutase) and Ole e 9 (1,3-β-glucanase). The anti-Ole e 1 mAb was kindly provided by Dr. Carlos Lahoz (Fundación Jiménez Díaz, Madrid, Spain) (Lauzurica et al. 1988). The anti-Ole e 2 polyclonal antibody (PoAb) was produced by immunization of rabbits with a keyhole limpet hemocyanin (KLH)-linked synthetic peptide (AQSATFPQFKPEEM) designed from the predicted amino acid sequence of an olive profilin (Ole e 2). Specificity of the antibody was already reported by Western blotting experiments and immunolocalization of the allergen (Morales et al. 2008). The anti-Ole e 9 polyclonal Ab was produced as described above using a synthetic peptide (YPYFAYKNQPTPDT) from the Ole e 9 amino acid sequence (Huecas et al. 2001; Duffort et al. 2006). Finally, we also purchased a commercially available PoAb that recognizes a chloroplastidic isoform of Cu/Zn-superoxide dismutase (SOD) from *Arabidopsis thaliana* (Agrisera, city, Sweden, Product No AS06 170), with probed cross-reactivity to Ole e 5 (Zafra 2007).

Primary Abs were diluted in blocking solution and incubated for 2 h at room temperature, whereas secondary Abs were diluted in TBST buffer and incubated for 1 h at room temperature in the dark. After Ab incubation, membranes were rinsed in TBST buffer four times for 5 min each. The different Abs used in this work and their corresponding dilutions are summarized in Table 1. Each experiment described below was repeated in triplicate. Negative controls included preimmune serum in the cases of Ole e 2 and Ole e 9.

Target	Primary antibody	Dilution	Secondary antibody	Dilution
Ole e 1	Mouse anti-olive Ole e 1 mAb (Lauzurica et al. 1988)	1:20,000	Goat anti-mouse IgG Ab, Alexa fluor 488-conjugated (Molecular Probes)	1:10,000
Ole e 2	Rabbit anti-olive Ole e 2 PoAb (Morales et al. 2008)	1:20,000	Donkey anti-rabbit IgG (Fab fragment) Ab, Cy3-conjugated (Jackson ImmunoResearch)	1:10,000
Ole e 5	Rabbit anti-Cu/Zn SOD PoAb (Agrisera Prod. No. AS06 170)	1:250	Goat anti-rabbit IgG Ab, Alexa fluor 633-conjugated (Molecular Probes)	1:10,000
Ole e 9 (N- domain)	Rabbit anti-olive Ole e 9 PoAb	1:10,000	Goat anti-rabbit IgG Ab, Alexa fluor 633-conjugated (Molecular Probes)	1:10,000

Table 1. Antibodies and dilutions used for immunoblotting experiments. mAb: monoclonal antibody; PoAb: polyclonal antibody.

Imaging was carried out with a Pharos FX Plus Molecular Imager (Bio-Rad) using the Quantity One v4.6.2 software (Bio-Rad).

2.4. Absolute and relative quantitation of allergens

The intensity of each fluorescent band was calculated using the quantitation tools of the Quantity One v4.6.2 software. In order to increase sensitivity of measurements and to avoid disturbing factors like the intensity of the background, the presence of individual non-specific spots, etc., two different methods for quantitation were used:

- For each allergen studied, reactive bands were identified, their optical density individually measured and then their absolute values added for each cultivar. Relative percentages of each allergen were then calculated for each cultivar, taking the cultivar with the highest optical density as the reference, which was assigned 100%.
- Simultaneous measurement of the optical density corresponding to all reactive bands from a given allergen in each cultivar was also performed. As before, relative percentages were also calculated, referred to the cultivar with the highest optical density, which was assigned 100%.

Finally, average of the percentages calculated by both methods was worked out, and the resulting percentages were newly made relative to the cultivar with the highest percentage, which was re-assigned 100%.

3. Results

3.1. SDS-PAGE protein profiles

Figure 1 shows the protein profiles of the extracts analysed after SDS-PAGE and Coomassie staining. The patterns observed for the major protein species were somewhat similar for all the cultivars tested. However, clear quantitative differences were distinguished, from which the most conspicuous were those in the protein range of 17-20 kDa. Proteins within this range were relatively abundant in the extracts corresponding to the cvs. 'Picual', 'Manzanilla', 'Cornicabra', 'Hojiblanca', 'Loaime', 'Blanqueta' and 'Lucio'.

When the commercial pollen extract was assayed by SDS-PAGE, a protein profile similar to the profile corresponding to the individual cultivars was observed, although several bands were absent or poorly resolved. Proteins in the range 17-20 kDa represented a low proportion of the total protein for this extract.

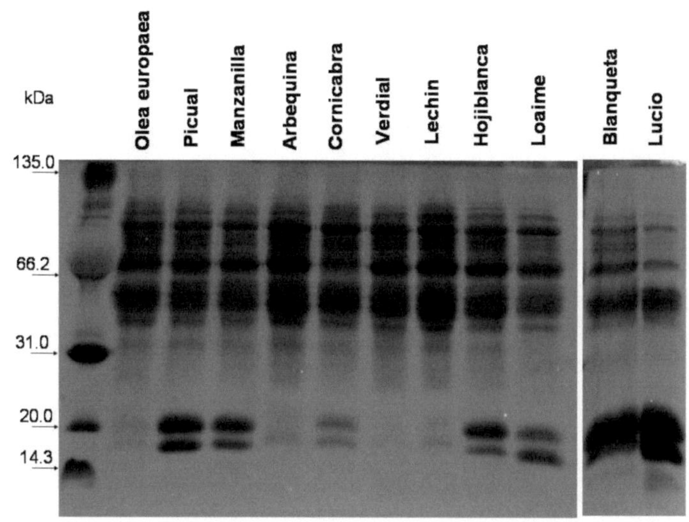

Figure 1. Coomassie stained SDS-PAGE gel of the univarietal pollen extracts and the commercial extract (*Olea europaea*) after using denaturing, reducing conditions. Gels contained 30 μg total protein per lane.

3.2. Immunoblot detection and quantitation of Ole e 1

Immunoblots probed with the monoclonal antibody to Ole e 1 resulted in the presence of two major immunoreactive bands of 18 and 20 kDa, corresponding to the monomeric non-glycosylated and mono-glycosylated forms (Figure 2). Other immunoreactive bands with low quantitative relevance were observed (36, 40 y 44 kDa) in several lanes.

Bands corresponding to the Mw of 18 and 20 kDa were quantitated according to the methods described above. Absolute measurements of the intensity of each individual band and both bands simultanously are displayed in Table 2, as well as the relative percentages calculated as described above.

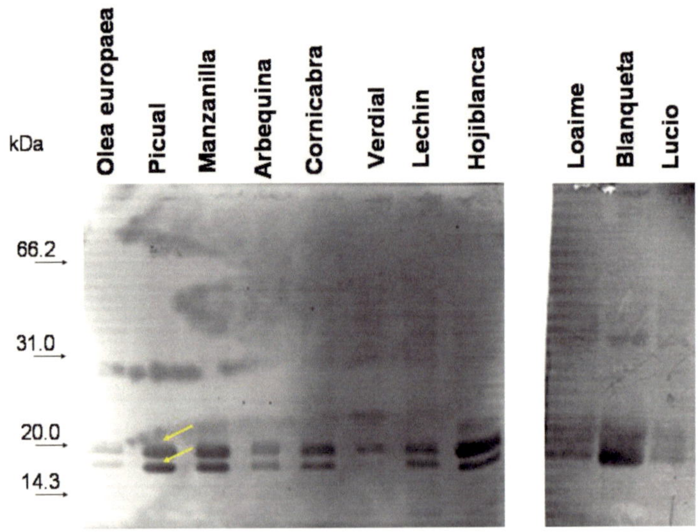

Figure 2. Immunoblot probed with the anti-Ole e 1 monoclonal antibody. Two major bands were observed (yellow arrows), corresponding to apparent molecular weights of 18 and 20 kDa.

	O. europaea	*Picual*	*Manzanilla*	*Arbequina*	*Cornicabra*	*Verdial*	*Lechín*	*Hojiblanca*	*Loaime*	*Blanqueta*	*Lucio*
18 kDa	3672	14385	16746	11894	20033	12174	17668	30706	41345	40388	17436
20 kDa	2348	10666	11233	7983	11716	3204	11804	22780	21143	32768	13087
Σ 18 and 20 kDa	6021	25051	27979	19877	31749	15378	29472	52784	62489	73156	30523
Relative %	8.23	34.24	38.25	27.17	43.40	21.02	40.28	72.15	85.41	100	41.72
18 and 20 kDa	6659	26741	29626	22044	34260	20950	32493	54095	60906	73900	30345
Relative %	9.01	36.18	40.09	29.83	46.36	28.35	43.97	73.21	82.42	100	41.06
Average relative %	8.62	35.21	39.17	28.5	41.88	24.68	42.125	72.68	83.915	100	41.39

Table 2. Quantitation of the two major bands cross-reactive to the anti Ole e 1 antibody. Absolute data in volume units (INT*mm^2).

3.3. Immunoblot detection and quantitation of Ole e 2

Immunoblots probed with the polyclonal antiserum to Ole e 2 resulted in the presence of up to five major immunoreactive bands of c.a. 14, 13.7, 14.2, 14.9 and 15.7 kDa (Figure 3).

Bands corresponding to the five Mws were quantitated according to the methods described above. Absolute measurements of the intensity of each individual band and all five bands simultanously are displayed in Table 3, as well as the relative percentages calculated as described above.

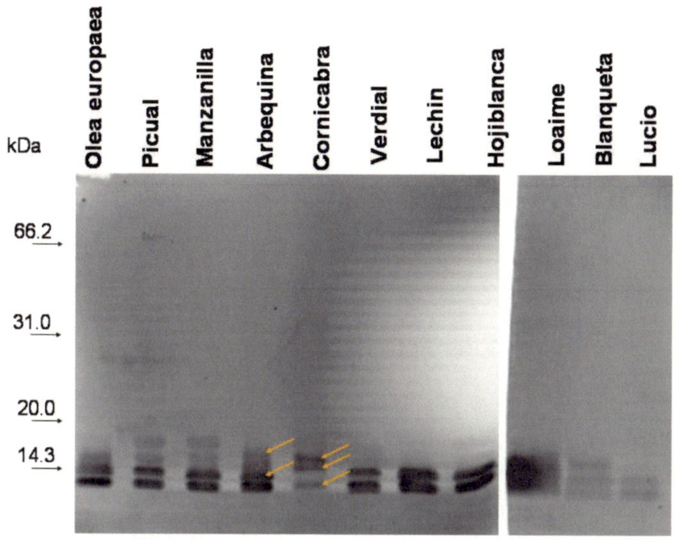

Figure 3. Immunoblot probed with the anti-Ole e 2 polyclonal antiserum. Five major bands were observed (orange arrows), corresponding to apparent molecular weights of 14, 13.7, 14.2, 14.9 and 15.7 kDa.

	O. europaea	*Picual*	*Manzanilla*	*Arbequina*	*Cornicabra*	*Verdial*	*Lechín*	*Hojiblanca*	*Loaime*	*Blanqueta*	*Lucio*
13.0 kDa	357152	277747	248153	405554	165942	394519	537187	356024	910640	476889	350778
13.7 kDa	398025	305569	261364	312528	198300*	250846	484703	463371	1004748	454397	486318
14.2 kDa	264210	198300*	198300*	223593	147305	198300*	198300*	198300*	987772	410790	198300*
14.9 kDa	198300*	198300*	198300*	198300*	290636	198300*	198300*	198300*	198300*	198300*	198300*
15.7 kDa	198300*	198300*	198300*	217632	198300*	198300*	198300*	198300*	198300*	198300*	198300*
Σ bands above	1415987	1178216	1104417	1357607	1000483	1240265	1616790	1414295	3299760	1738676	1431996
Relative %	42.91	35.70	33.47	41.14	30.31	37.59	49	42.86	100	52.70	43.39
All bands	2281004	2385713	2464789	2550651	2499993	2472138	2437099	2312637	2913894	2092950	1973168
Relative %	78.3	81.87	84.59	87.53	85.80	84.84	83.64	79.37	100	71.83	67.71
Average relative %	60.605	58.78	59.03	64.335	58.055	61.215	66.32	61.115	100	62.265	55.55

Table 3. Quantitation of the five major bands cross-reactive to the anti Ole e 2 antibody. Absolute data in volume units (INT*mm^2). *: band not present. The indicated value corresponds to the average of 5 measurements made in the background.

3.4. Immunoblot detection and quantitation of Ole e 5 and Ole e 9

Immunoblots probed with the commercial antibody to Cu,Zn SOD (Ole e 5) and the polyclonal antiserum to Ole e 9 resulted in the presence of up to five major immunoreactive bands of c.a. 16, 16.5, 22, 26 and 50 kDa for Ole e 5, and two immunoreactive bands of c.a. 36 and 46.5 kDa for Ole e 9 (Figure 4).

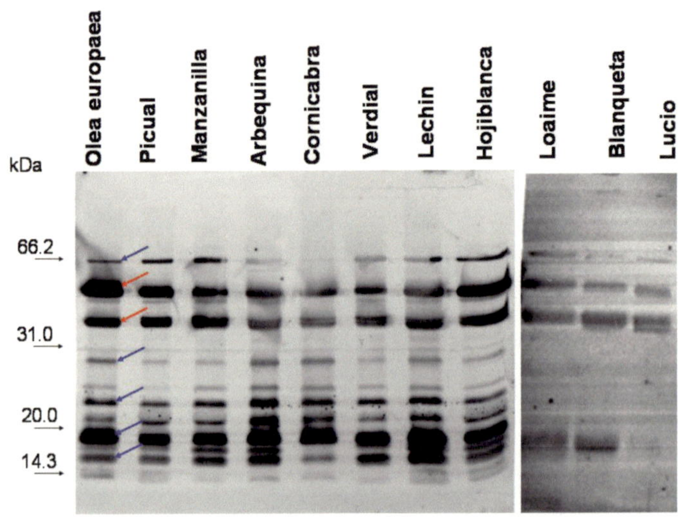

Figure 4. Immunoblot probed with the anti- Cu,Zn-SOD (Ole e 5) commercial antibody and the polyclonal antiserum to Ole e 9. Five major bands were observed (blue arrows), corresponding to apparent molecular weights of 16, 16.5, 22, 26 and 50 kDa for Ole e 5, and two immunoreactive bands of c.a. 36 and 46.5 kDa for Ole e 9 (red arrows).

Bands corresponding to the five Mws of Ole e 5 and two of Ole e 9 were quantitated according to the methods described above. Absolute measurements of the intensity of each individual band and all five bands simultanously are displayed in Tables 4 and 5, as well as the relative percentages calculated as described above.

4. Clustering of cultivars according to their relative allergenic content

Table 6 summarizes the final relative averages of reactivity calculated for each cultivar and allergen. Relative values present a wide range in the case of allergens Ole e 1 and Ole e 9, whereas Ole e 2 and Ole e 5 allergens maintain values relatively constant, higher than 50% for all cultivars, with a single exception (Ole e 5 in the cultivar 'Lucio').

Therefore, the following thresholds have been defined in order to divide cultivars into cultivars with high/average/low allergenic content for the allergens Ole e 1 and Ole e 9. In the case of Ole e 1, we have considered that percentages of 30% and 35% may represent reasonable limits, taking into account the extremely high content of some cultivars in this allergen, which may represents up to 23% of the total protein content for these cultivars (Castro et al. 2003). For Ole e 9, the percentages of 40% and 60% were selected as the thresholds.

	O. europaea	*Picual*	*Manzanilla*	*Arbequina*	*Cornicabra*	*Verdial*	*Lechín*	*Hojiblanca*	*Loaime*	*Blanqueta*	*Lucio*
16.0 kDa	12522	10472	13810	16174	8515	16875	20320	19682	1054	793	714
16.5 kDa	33503	21491	23191	27710	33630	28904	36422	39682	27218	23811	4304
22.0 kDa	9451	7946	9623	14385	12453	9703	13812	17211	6380	5201	5041
26.0 kDa	6221	3389	3688	7134	7617	4447	7775	11424	12698	9191	7098
50.0 kDa	5611	7474	9643	4818	3941	5794	8238	19507	12979	5625	4200
Σ bands above	67308	50772	59955	70221	66156	65723	86567	107506	47350	44621	21357
Relative %	62.61	47.23	55.77	65.32	61.54	61.13	80.52	100	44.04	41.51	19.87
All bands	122909	95529	107694	136847	128879	118503	157103	155113	136354	107779	79135
Relative %	78.23	60.81	68.55	87.11	82.03	75.43	100	98.73	86.79	68.60	50.37
Average relative %	70.42	54.02	62.16	76.215	71.785	68.28	90.26	99.365	65.415	55.055	35.12
Average relative to 100 %	70.87	54.36	62.55	76.70	72.24	68.72	90.83	100	65.83	55.41	**35.34**

Table 4. Quantitation of the five major bands cross-reactive to the anti Cu,Zn SOD (Ole e 5) antibody. Absolute data in volume units (INT*mm²). In this case, the average relative percentage was again referred to 100%, as the maximun relative percentages previously calculated corresponded to two different cultivars ('Hojiblanca' and 'Lechín').

	O. europaea	*Picual*	*Manzanilla*	*Arbequina*	*Cornicabra*	*Verdial*	*Lechín*	*Hojiblanca*	*Loaime*	*Blanqueta*	*Lucio*
36 kDa	20241	18902	25868	18912	15583	17605	24746	44273	29766	28377	20736
46.5 kDa	39567	23419	17751	16764	13584	13916	20517	53338	22784	13160	12730
Σ 36 and 46.5 kDa	59808	42322	43619	35677	29167	31521	45264	97612	52550	41538	33467
Relative %	61.27	43.36	44.68	36.55	29.88	32.29	46.37	100	53.83	42.55	34.28
36 and 46.5 kDa	72676	51950	56389	47169	39589	45075	59672	102195	74531	52213	39717
Relative %	71.11	50.83	55.17	46.15	38.73	44.10	58.39	100	72.93	51.09	38.86
Average relative %	66.19	47.095	49.925	41.35	34.305	38.195	52.38	100	63.38	46.82	36.57

Table 5. Quantitation of the two major bands cross-reactive to the anti Ole e 9 antibody. Absolute data in volume units (INT*mm²).

	O. europaea	*Picual*	*Manzanilla*	*Arbequina*	*Cornicabra*	*Verdial*	*Lechín*	*Hojiblanca*	*Loaime*	*Blanqueta*	*Lucio*	*Thresholds low/average/high*
Ole e 1	8.62	35.21	39.17	28.5	41.88	24.68	42.125	72.68	83.915	100	41.39	30%-35%
Ole e 2	60.605	58.78	59.03	64.335	58.055	61.215	66.32	61.115	100	62.265	55.55	-
Ole e 5	70.87	54.36	62.55	76.70	72.24	68.72	90.83	100	65.83	55.41	35.34	-
Ole e 9	66.19	47.095	49.925	41.35	34.305	38.195	52.38	100	63.38	46.82	36.57	40%-60%

Table 6. Abstract of the relative percentages of reactivity corresponding to the cultivars analysed for each allergen. High reactivity is marked by using bold text, and low reactivity is marked by italics, after considering the thresholds indicated.

The following categories were established after following the above mentioned criteria:

- 'Hojiblanca'-type extract, characterized by high contents of Ole e 1 and Ole e 9. The cultivar 'Loaime' could be included in this same group.
- 'Picual'- type extract, characterized by high content of Ole e 1 and low to average contents of Ole e 9. The cultivars 'Manzanilla', 'Lucio', 'Cornicabra', 'Lechín' and 'Blanqueta' could be included in this same group.
- 'Arbequina' -type extract, characterized by low content in both Ole e 1 and Ole e 9, with average to high contents of Ole e 5 and Ole e 2. The cultivar 'Verdial' could be included in this same group.

The *Olea europaea* commercial extract doesn't match any of the tested cultivars, corresponding to an extract with a relative high proportion of Ole e 9 and low proportion of Ole e 1.

This initial proposal should be implemented by further analyzing additional olive pollen allergens (some of them highly relevant from a clinical point of view like Ole e 7), and by analyzing the allergen profiles of other agronomically relevant cultivars. However, the classification obtained here is in good agreement with the genetic relationships among cultivars already described on the basis of Ole e 1 and Ole e 2 polymorphism (Hamman-Khalifa et al. 2008; Jiménez-López et al., 2012). Moreover, this classification also supports clinical findings describing sharp differences in patient's reactivity to commercially available extracts depending on their place of residence in Spain, where these model cultivars are differentially predominant (Casanovas et al. 1997). Providing that sensitization to specific allergens can be determined in individual patients, the application of the concept of allergenic profile to allergen extracts could be considered a major adventage. This concept would therefore open the posibility of choosing the allergen extract matching the sensitivity of each patient. Moreover, the continuous development of new molecular tools (e.g. new antibodies with higher specificity) will undoubtedly improve the present type of studies, which has to be considered still preliminary.

Acknowledgements

This work was supported by the Spanish Ministry of Science and Innovation (MICINN) (ERDF-cofinanced projects AGL2008-00517, BFU2011-22779 and PIE-200840I186) and the Junta de Andalucía (ERDF-cofinanced projects P2010-CVI5767 and P2010-AGR6274). The authors acknowledge the availability of plant material and the collaboration of the staff of the IFAPA center "Venta del Llano" (Mengíbar, Spain) depending from the Andalusian Regional Government.

Author details

Sonia Morales, Antonio Jesús Castro, Carmen Salmerón,
María Isabel Rodríguez-García and Juan de Dios Alché
Estación Experimental del Zaidín (CSIC), Granada, Spain

Francisco Manuel Marco
R&D Inmunal S.A.U. Tecnoalcalá, Alcalá de Henares, Madrid, Spain

Sonia Morales
Proteomic Research Service, Hospital Universitario San Cecilio, Granada, Spain

5. References

Alché, J.D., Castro, A.J., Jiménez-López, J.C., Morales, S., Zafra, A., Hamman-Khalifa, A.M. & Rodríguez-García, M.I. (2007). Differential characteristics of olive pollen from different cultivars: biological and clinical implications. *Journal of Investigational Allergology & Clinical Immunology*, Vol. 17, Suppl 1., pp. 63-68, ISSN 1018-9068

Alché, J.D., Castro, A.J., Olmedilla, A., Fernández, M.C., Rodríguez, R., Villalba, M. & Rodríguez-García, M.I. (1999). The major olive pollen allergen (Ole e I) shows both gametophytic and sporophytic expression during anther development, and its synthesis and storage takes place in the RER. *Journal of Cell Science*, Vol. 112, No. 15, pp. 2501-2509, ISSN 0021-9533

Alché, J.D., Cismondi, I.D., Castro, A.J., Hamman Khalifa, A., & Rodríguez García, M.I. (2003). Temporal and spatial gene expression of Ole e 3 allergen in olive (*Olea europaea* L.) pollen. *Acta Biologica Cracoviensia, Series Botanica*, Vol. 45, No. 1, pp. 89-95, ISSN 0001-5296

Alché, J.D., Corpas, F., Rodríguez-García, M.I., & del Río, L.A. (1998). Identification and immunolocalization of superoxide dismutase isoenzymes of olive pollen. *Physiologia Plantarum*, Vol. 104, No. 4, pp. 772-776, ISSN 1399-3054

Alché, J.D., M'rani-Alaoui, M., Castro, A.J., & Rodríguez-García, M.I. (2004). Ole e 1, the major allergen from olive (*Olea europaea* L.) pollen, increases its expression and is released to the culture medium during in vitro germination. *Plant & Cell Physiology*, Vol. 45, No. 9, pp. 1149-1157, ISSN 0032-0781

Alché, J.D., Rodríguez-García, M.I., Castro, A.J., & Alché, V. (2005). Kit para el diagnóstico de hipersensibilidad frente a alergenos del polen del olivo y su utilización. *Spanish Office for Patents Bulletin* (OEPM). Publication reference 2 196 952.

Alché, J.D., Rodríguez-García, M.I., Castro, A.J., & Alché, V. (2010). Perfeccionamientos introducidos en el objeto de solicitud de patente española Nº P200100995. *Spanish Office for Patents Bulletin* (OEPM). Publication reference 2 326 399.

Asturias, J.A., Arilla, M.C., Gómez-Bayon, N., Martínez, J., Martínez, A., & Palacios, R. (1997). Cloning and expression of the panallergen profilin and the major allergen (Ole e 1) from olive tree pollen. *Journal of Allergy & Clinical Immunology*, Vol. 100, No. 3, pp. 365-372, ISSN 0091-6749

Barranco, D., Trujillo, I., & Rallo, L. (2005). Libro I. Elaiografía Hispánica. In: Variedades del olivo en España. Rallo, L., Barranco, D., Caballero, J.M., Del Río, C., Martín, A., Tous, J., & Trujillo, I. (Eds.) Madrid: Junta de Andalucía, MAPA and Ediciones Mundi-prensa.

Carnés Sánchez, J., Iraola, V.M., Sastre, J., Florido, F., Boluda, L., & Fernández-Caldas, E. (2002). Allergenicity and immunochemical characterization of six varieties of Olea europaea. *Allergy*, Vol. 57, No. 4, pp. 313-318, ISSN 0105-4538

Casanovas, M., Florido, F., Sáenz de San Pedro, B., González, P., Martínez-Alzamora, F., Marañón, F., & Fernández-Caldas, E. (1977). Sensitization to Olea europaea: geographical differences and discrepancies. *Allergologia et Immunopathologia (Madrid)*, Vol. 25, No. 4, pp. 159-166

Castro, A.J., Alché, J.D., Cuevas, J., Romero, P.J., Alché, V., & Rodríguez-García, M.I. (2003). Pollen from different olive tree cultivars contains varying amounts of the major allergen Ole e 1. *International Archives of Allergy & Immunology*, Vol. 131, No. 3, pp. 164-173, ISSN 1018-2438

Castro, A.J., Bednarczyk, A., Schaeffer-Reiss, C., Rodríguez-García, M.I. Van Dorsselaer, A., & Alché, J.D. (2010). Screening of Ole e 1 polymorphism among olive cultivars by peptide mapping and N-glycopeptide analysis. *Proteomics*, Vol. 10, pp. 953-962, ISSN 1615-9861

Conde Hernández, J., Conde Hernández, P., González Quevedo Tejerina, M.T., Conde Alcañiz, M.A., Conde Alcañiz, E.M., Crespo Moreira, P., & Cabanillas Platero, M. (2002). Antigenic and allergenic differences between 16 different cultivars of Olea europaea. *Allergy*, Vol. 57 Suppl. 71, pp. 60-65, ISSN 0105-4538

Duffort, O., Palomares, O., Lombardero, M., Villalba, M., Barber, D., Rodríguez, R., & Polo, F. (2006). Variability of Ole e 9 Allergen in Olive Pollen Extracts: Relevance of Minor Allergens in Immunotherapy Treatments. *International Archives of Allergy & Immunology*, Vol. 140, No. 2, pp. 131-138, ISSN 1018-2438

Fernández-Caldas, E., Carnés, J., Iraola, V., & Casanovas, M. (2007). Comparison of the allergenicity and Ole e 1 content of 6 varieties of Olea euroapea pollen collected during 5 consecutive years. *Annals of Allergy, Asthma & Immunology*, Vol. 98, No. 5, pp. 464-470, ISSN 1081-1206

Geller-Bernstein, C., Arad, G., Keynan, N., Lahoz, C., Cardaba, B., & Waisel, Y. (1996). Hypersensitivity to pollen of Olea europaea in Israel. *Allergy*, Vol. 51, No. 5, pp. 356-359, ISSN 0105-4538

Hamman-Khalifa, A.M. (2005). Utilización de marcadores relacionados con la alergenicidad y la biosíntesis de lípidos para la discriminación entre cultivares de olivo. *Ph.D. report. University of Granada*. Spain.

Hamman-Khalifa, A.M., Alché, J.D., & Rodríguez-García, M.I. (2003). Discriminación molecular en el polen de variedades españolas y marroquíes de olivo (Olea europaea L.). *Polen*, Vol. 13, pp. 219-225, ISSN 1135-8408

Hamman Khalifa, A.M., Castro, A.J., Rodríguez García, M.I., & Alché, J.D (2008). Olive cultivar origin is a major cause of polymorphism for Ole e 1 pollen allergen. *BMC Plant Biology*, Vol. 8, pp. 10, ISSN 1471-2229

Huecas, S., Villalba, M., & Rodríguez, R. (2001). Ole e 9, a major olive pollen allergen is a 1,3-beta-glucanase. Isolation, characterization, amino acid sequence, and tissue specificity. *Journal of Biological Chemistry*, Vol. 276, No. 30, pp. 27959-27966, ISSN 0021-9258

Jiménez-López, J.C. (2008). Caracterización molecular del polimorfismo de las profilinas en el polen del olivo y otras especies alergogénicas. *Ph. D. report. University of Granada*. Spain.

Jiménez-López, J.C., Morales, S., Castro, A.J., Volkmann, D., Rodríguez-García, M.I. & Alché, J.D. (2012). Characterization of profilin polymorphism in pollen with a focus on multifunctionality. *PLoS One*, Vol. 7, No. 2, p. e30878, ISSN 1932-6203

Lauzurica, P., Gurbindo, C., Maruri, N., Galocha, B., Díaz, R., González, J., García, R. & Lahoz, C. (1988). Olive (*Olea europaea*) pollen allergens. I. Immunochemical characterization by immunoblotting, CRIE and immunodetection by a monoclonal antibody. *Molecular Immunology*, Vol. 25, pp. 329-335, ISSN 0161-5890

Liccardi, G., D'Amato, M., & D'Amato, G. (1996). Oleaceae pollinosis: a review. *International Archives of Allergy & Immunology*, Vol. 111, No. 3, pp. 210-217, ISSN 1018-2438

Lombardero, M., Barbas, J.A., Moscoso del Prado, J., & Carreira J. (1994). cDNA sequence analysis of the main olive allergen, Ole e I. *Clinical & Experimental Allergy*, Vol. 24, No. 8, pp. 765-770, ISSN 1365-2222

Martínez, A., Asturias, J.A., Monteseirín, J., Moreno, V., García-Cubillana, A., Hernández, M., de la Calle, A., Sánchez-Hernández, C., Pérez-Formoso, J.L., & Conde, J. (2002). The allergenic relevance of profilin (Ole e 2) from *Olea europaea* pollen. *Allergy*, Vol. 57, Suppl. 71, pp. 17-23, ISSN 0105-4538

Morales, S., Castro, A.J., Jiménez-López, J.C., Florido, F., Rodríguez-García, M.I., & Alché J.D. (2012). A novel multiplex method for the simultaneous detection and relative quantification of pollen allergens. *Electrophoresis,* Vol. 33, pp. 1-8, DOI 10.1002/elps.201100667, ISSN: 1522-2683

Morales, S., Jiménez-López, J.C., Castro, A.J., Rodríguez-García, M.I., & Alché, J.D. (2008). Olive pollen profilin (Ole e 2 allergen) co-localizes with highly active areas of the actin cytoskeleton and is released to the culture medium during in vitro pollen germination. *Journal of Microscopy-Oxford*, Vol. 231, No. 2, pp. 332-341, ISSN 1365-2818

Tejera, M.L., Villalba, M., Batanero, E., & Rodríguez, R. (1999). Identification, isolation, and characterization of Ole e 7, a new allergen of olive tree pollen. *The Journal of Allergy & Clinical Immunology*, Vol. 104, No. 4, pp. 797-802, ISSN 0091-6749

Villalba, M., Batanero, E., Lopez-Otín, C., Sánchez, L.M., Monsalve, R.I., González de la Peña, M.A., Lahoz, C., & Rodríguez, R. (1993). The amino acid sequence of Ole e I, the major allergen from olive tree (*Olea europaea*) pollen. *European Journal of Biochemistry*, Vol. 216, No. 3, pp. 863-869, ISSN 0014-2956

Villalba, M., Batanero, E., Monsalve, R.I., González de la Peña, M.A. Lahoz, C., & Rodríguez, R. (1994). Cloning and expression of Ole e I, the major allergen from olive tree pollen. Polymorphism analysis and tissue specificity. *Journal of Biological Chemistry*, Vol. 269, No. 21, pp. 15217-15222, ISSN 0021-9258

Wheeler, A.W. (1992). Hypersensitivity to the allergens of the pollen from the olive tree (Olea europaea). *Clinical and Experimental Allergy*, Vol. 22, No. 12, pp. 1052-1057, ISSN 1365-2222

Zafra, A. (2007). Caracterización preliminar del polimorfismo de la proteína alergénica Ole e 5 en el polen del olivo de distintos cultivares. *Master Thesis. University of Granada.* Spain.

Chapter 3

Detection and Quantitation of Olive Pollen Allergen Isoforms Using 2-D Western Blotting

Krzysztof Zienkiewicz, Estefanía García-Quirós, Juan de Dios Alché, María Isabel Rodríguez-García and Antonio Jesús Castro

Additional information is available at the end of the chapter

http://dx.doi.org/10.5772/46171

1. Introduction

The use of biological extracts for allergy diagnosis and immunotherapy has some disadvantages, including the high variability in their allergenic composition and the presence of allergens to which the patient is not allergic. As the result, wrong diagnosis, new sensitizations and/or systemic reactions often occur, limiting their use for specific immunotherapy. One of the strategies to overcome these problems is the standardization of biological extracts in order to control their allergenic composition. For this purpose, it is highly recommended to identify the allergenic molecules in the extract, to quantify them and to evaluate their allergenic activity in sensitized patients.

The allergenic pollen used for the preparation of natural extracts or recombinant allergens may contain different allergenic isoforms and/or variable amounts of each allergen, depending of its genetic origin among other factors (Castro et al. 2003, Hamman-Khalifa et al. 2008, Castro et al. 2010 & Jiménez-López et al. 2012). Consequently, allergic patients from different geographical areas may exhibit differential sensitization to a given allergen (Movérare et al. 2002). This fact can hinder the diagnosis of an allergic patient in response to a particular extract. Therefore, the allergenic variability in standardized protein extracts should resemble as much as possible to that observed in the natural sources in order to assure the efficiency and safety in the diagnosis and immunotherapy procedures.

Olive pollen produces seasonal respiratory allergy in the Mediterranean area, as well as in other temperate regions where it is intensively cultivated. Eleven olive pollen allergens, called Ole e 1 to Ole e 11, have been identified and characterized so far (Esteve et al. 2012). Many of these proteins exhibit a significant polymorphism as a consequence of the existence of point substitutions in the amino acid sequence, posttranslational modifications (e.g. glycosylation), and/or multimeric forms (Castro et al. 2010). In addition, some allergens show major quantitative differences, depending on the genetic origin (i.e. cultivar) of pollen (Castro et al. 2003). Here, we have used a 2-D electrophoresis-based immunodetection method to analyze the molecular variability of four olive allergens, namely Ole e 1, Ole e 2, Ole e 7 and Ole e 9, in the pollen of the olive cultivar 'Picual'. The advantages and putative applications of this method are also discussed.

2. Polymorphism of olive pollen allergens

The olive (*Olea europaea* L.) pollen exhibits a complex allergenic profile with numerous proteins recognized by sera of olive pollen allergic patients (Rodríguez et al. 2002 & Esteve et al. 2012). The great majority of olive pollen allergens show a highly polymorphic nature in 1-D and 2-D polyacrylamide gels, resulting in a pattern of multiple bands or spots, respectively.

Ole e 1 is the main olive pollen allergen, and affects more than 70% of patients suffering from olive pollinosis. Ole e 1 is an acidic protein that consists of a single 145 amino acid polypeptide chain, which is glycosylated at Asn^{111} (Lombardero et al. 1992). The molecular function of Ole e 1 is unknown but, on the basis of its cellular location and expression pattern, it has been suggested that it might have a role in pollen-pistil communication during pollen tube growth (Alché et al. 1999 & Alché et al. 2004). After 1-D SDS-PAGE and staining, or blotting and immunolabeling with specific antibodies or sera from allergic patients, three bands of 18.5, 20, and 22 kDa are visible, corresponding to the non-glycosylated, glycosylated and hyperglycosylated Ole e 1 isoforms, respectively (Villalba et al. 1993). Under non-reducing running conditions, a dimeric form of 40 kDa has been also detected (Villalba et al. 1993 & Morales et al. 2012). Ole e 1 is highly polymorphic due to the presence of point changes in the nucleotide sequence. These changes are extended to the expressed protein, affecting up to 59 different positions in the amino acid sequence (Villalba et al. 1994, Hamman-Khalifa et al. 2008 & Castro et al. 2010). Some of these amino acid substitutions are located within the epitope sequences involved in IgG and IgE binding (González et al. 2002). The composition of the sugar moiety is also highly variable among allergen isoforms (Castro et al. 2010). Interestingly, the N-linked glycan contributes to the final immunogenic and allergenic capacity of Ole e 1 (Batanero et al. 1994, 1999). The varietal origin of pollen represents a major source of variability for Ole e 1 (Hamman-Khalifa et al. 2008 & Castro et al. 2010). Moreover, this allergen showed conspicuous quantitative differences among olive cultivars (Castro et al. 2003).

Ole e 2 allergen belongs to the profilin family. Profilins are ubiquitous proteins, which are present in all eukaryotic cells. They control actin polymerization (Karlsson and Lindberg 2007), being key mediators of the membrane–cytoskeleton communication (Baluska and Volkmann 2002). As allergens, profilins have been identified in various plant sources, such as pollen, latex, fruits and vegetables (Santos and Van Ree 2011). They have been designed as panallergens since they are responsible for many IgE cross-reactions between unrelated pollen and plant food allergenic sources (Valenta et al. 1992 & Santos and Van Ree 2011). Ole 2 has a clinical prevalence of 24% in the allergic population (Asturias et al. 1997,

Ledesma et al. 1998a, Martínez et al. 2002 & Quiralte et al. 2007). Four Ole e 2 isoforms of 17.8, 17.0, 16.0, and 15.2 kDa were firstly determined (Asturias et al. 1997). Three isoforms with molecular weights of 13.3, 13.9 and 14.3 kDa are distinguishable after 1-D SDS-PAGE in the 'Picual' pollen (Morales et al. 2008). Two additional isoforms with apparent molecular masses of 15.7 and 14.9 kDa have been described in the cultivar 'Verdial de Huévar' (Alché et al. 2007). Under non-reducing electrophoretic conditions, a dimer form of Ole e 2 of about 32 kDa has been identified (Ledesma et al. 1998a). Recently, the polymorphism of the allergen Ole e 2 was evaluated in 24 olive cultivars (Jiménez-López et al. 2012). Data showed that profilins displayed 28.2 and 24.6% of variability among cultivars for nucleotide and amino acid sequences, respectively. Ole e 2 sequences had 130, 131 or 134 amino acids length and 39 amino acid positions were variable among the cultivars analyzed.

Ole e 3 and Ole e 8 allergens are Ca^{2+}-binding proteins involved in intracellular signalling processes (Batanero et al. 1996b & Ledesma et al. 1998b, 2000). Ole e 3 is a small (9.2 kDa) and acidic (pI 4.2-4.3) protein, which is specifically expressed in pollen (Ledesma et al. 1998b & Alché et al. 2003). It belongs to a new Ca^{2+}-binding protein subfamily named polcalcins (Ledesma et al. 1998b), which has also been established as a new panallergen. The allergenic activity of polcalcins is primarily associated with the Ca^{2+}-bound isoforms (Engel et al. 1997, Hayek et al. 1998 & Twardosz et al. 1997). The prevalence of Ole e 3 is higher than 50% of the olive pollen sensitized population (Batanero et al. 1996a). This allergen shows polymorphism at positions 43 ($L \leftrightarrow P$) and 80 ($V \leftrightarrow I$) of its amino acid sequence (Ledesma et al. 1998b). Ole e 8 consists of a single polypeptide of 20 kDa and its clinical incidence is as low as 3-4% (Ledesma et al. 2002). The molecular variability of Ole e 8 remains to be studied.

Ole e 4 and Ole e 6 allergens have no homology with other known proteins. Ole e 4 has an IgE-binding frequency by immunoblot of 80% (Boluda et al. 1998), while the prevalence of Ole e 6 depends on the geographical zone and reaches values between 10 and 55% (Batanero et al. 1997). Ole e 4 consists of a single acidic polypeptide chain with an apparent molecular weight of 32 kDa, and at least two isoforms with pIs between 4.6 and 5.1 have been described (Boluda et al. 1998). Ole e 6 is a Cys-rich small protein of 5.8 kDa and its amino acid sequence shows no microheterogeneities (Batanero et al. 1997).

Ole e 5 is a CuZn-superoxide dismutase (SOD) with a molecular weight of 16 kDa, which catalyzes the dismutation of superoxide into oxygen and hydrogen peroxide, forming part of the cellular antioxidant defence system (Alché et al. 1998). This olive pollen allergen has an IgE-binding frequency of about 35% in the population assayed (Butteroni et al. 2005). Several studies have demonstrated that Ole e 5 shows a remarkable degree of polymorphism. Thus, the olive pollen of the variety 'Picual' contains at least 4 isoforms of the enzyme with pIs of 4.60, 4.78, 5.08, and 5.22, respectively (Alché et al. 1998). In addition, Boluda et al. (1998) described five isoforms with pIs between 5.1 and 6.5 in a commercial pollen sample of uncertain varietal origin from USA. More recently, Butteroni et al. (2005) reported discrepancies between the Ole e 5 amino acid sequences of the native and the recombinant forms.

Ole e 7 allergen exhibits a high homology with several lipid transfer proteins (LTPs). It is a small protein (10 kDa), which exhibits a high degree of polymorphism (Tejera et al. 1999). Thus, two isoforms with microheterogeneities at positions 4, 5, 10 and 11 of the N-terminal domain of the allergen have been described (Tejera et al. (1999). Ole e 7 is recognized by sera of 47% of patients allergic to olive pollen (Tejera et al. 1999). The ubiquitous nature of Ole e 7 and its high homology with LTPs from other plant species explains its high cross-reactivity and its designation as panallergen (Díaz-Perales et al. 2000).

Ole e 9 is a 1,3-β-glucanase and belongs to group 2 of pathogenesis-related proteins. This glycoprotein displays a molecular weight of 46.4 kDa on 1-D gels and is composed of two immunologically independent domains: an N-terminal domain (NtD) with 1,3-β-glucanase activity, and a C-terminal domain (CtD) that binds 1,3-β-glucans (Treviño et al. 2008). The clinical incidence of Ole e 9 is high, affecting the 65% of olive allergic patients. After SDS-PAGE under non-reducing conditions, a monomeric form of the allergen (46 kDa) and its dimer (91 kDa) are distinguishable. Ole e 9 shows a low but still significant level of polymorphism due to the presence of microheterogeneities in its amino acid sequence (Huecas et al. 2009). Thus, IEF analysis of the purified protein rendered four bands with pI values of 4.8, 4.9, 5.1, and 5.4 (Huecas et al. 2009). Ole e 9 has two potential N-glycosylation sites at positions Asn-355 and Asn-447. This N-linked sugar motif might also contribute to increase the molecular variability of Ole e 9, as it does for Ole e 1.

Ole e 10 is a small protein (10 kDa), which belongs to a new carbohydrate-binding-module (CBM43) family and binds specifically 1,3-β-glucans (Barral et al. 2005). The protein is composed of 102 amino acid residues and shows partial homology with the C-terminal domain of Ole e 9. Co-localization of Ole e 10 and callose in the growing pollen tube suggests a role for this protein in pollen tube wall remodelling during germination (Barral et al. 2005). Ole e 10 has been described as a major inducer of type I allergy in humans. It is involved in the allergic responses of 55% of patients suffering olive polinosis (Barral et al. 2005). However, there is no data about the polymorphism of this allergen so far.

Finally, Ole e 11 allergen is a pollen pectin methylesterase (PME) with an apparent molecular weight of 37.4 (Salamanca et al. 2010). PMEs are involved in demethylation of cell wall pectic compounds and they are key regulators of pollen tube growth (Bosch et al. 2005 & Jiang et al. 2005). The prevalence of this allergen between different populations of olive allergic patients varies from 55.9% to 75.6% (Salamanca et al. 2010). The molecular polymorphism of Ole e 11 remains to be studied.

The molecular variability of olive allergens is underrepresented in commercial protein extracts of olive pollen that are used for allergen-specific diagnosis and treatment of allergy (Morales et al. 2012). The relative abundance of individual isoforms with distinct IgE-reactivity within the protein content might affect the total allergenic potency of the extract. This, in turn, could lead to ambiguities in the IgE-binding responses detected for these allergens. Therefore, it is important to ensure that the allergenic variability in standardized protein extracts resembles as much as possible to that observed in the natural sources from which such extracts are prepared (Morales et al. 2012).

3. Immunoblotting as a tool for allergen standardization

The standardization of commercial olive pollen extracts is of great importance in order to assure efficiency and safety in the allergy diagnosis and immunotherapy procedures (Morales et al. 2012). Allergen standardization in European and United States legislations is mainly based on IgE-binding potencies and not on the content of individual allergens in a protein extract. Current procedures for preparation of protein extracts from natural sources are frequently inadequate, because they are standardized by determining the IgE response of a population, which is represented by a pool of sera from allergic patients, to major allergens present in these extracts (Morales et al. 2012). On the contrary, IgE binding to minor allergens will be difficult to detect because of their relatively low content in the extract. Thus, only major allergens will be considered in biological standardization (van Ree 1997, 2007). The most common allergy diagnostic tests can be performed *in vivo*, like SPT (Skin Prick Test), or *in vitro*, by competitive assays such as RAST (RadioAllergoSorbent Test) or ELISA (Enzyme-Linked ImmunoSorbent Assay). All these methods measure the total allergenic activity, but they do not explain the contribution of each individual allergen to the allergic response (Morales et al. 2012). Therefore, in addition to the allergenic potency of a protein extract, it is necessary to determine the molecular variability of these allergens. For this purpose, methods based on electrophoretic separation of proteins and immunoblotting are particularly useful and should be used in parallel to *in vitro* competitive assays (Baldo 1983). Thus, antibodies raised against specific allergens can be used to detect and quantify the different allergen isoforms present in non-standardized extracts. Such analysis can help, in turn, to design adequate dosage schemes and to elucidate the dose-therapeutic response of major and minor allergens.

3.1. Detection of olive pollen allergen isoforms by 2-D Western blotting

Protein extracts were prepared from mature pollen grains collected from olive (*Olea europaea* L.) trees (cv. 'Picual') grown in the province of Granada (Spain). Pollen samples (0.1 g) were suspended in 2.5 mL extraction buffer consisting of 40 mM Tris-HCl (pH 7.0), 2% (v/v) Triton X-100, 60 mM DTT, and 10 μL of a protease inhibitor cocktail (Sigma-Aldrich, St. Louis, MI, USA). Proteins were allowed to elute for 2 h at 4°C under continuous stirring. The resulting supernatants were desalted and delipidated in a PD-10 column (GE Healthcare Bio-Sciences AB, Uppsala, Sweden). Pollen proteins were then precipitated at −20°C for 1 h in a solution of 20% (w/v) trichloroacetic acid (TCA) prepared in acetone. The resulting pellet was resuspended in 0.5 mL solubilization buffer (7 M urea, 2 M thiourea, 4% w/v CHAPS, 5 mM tributylphosphine (TBP), 0.5% (v/v) Bio-Lyte 3–10 buffer (Bio-Rad, Hercules, CA, USA) and traces of bromophenol blue). Total protein content was estimated using the 2D Quant Kit (Amersham Biosciences, Piscataway, NJ, USA) according to the manufacturer's instructions.

Samples containing ~75 μg of total protein were applied to 7 cm polyacrylamide strips (pH 3–10NL, Bio-Rad) by in-gel rehydration at 30 V for 12 h. Focusing was conducted at 20°C in an Ettan IPGphor 3 Cell (GE Healthcare Bio-Sciences AB, Uppsala, Sweden) as follows: 300 and 1000 V for 1 h each followed by a linear increase from 1000 to 10,000 V, and finally 10,000 V to give a total of 40 kVh. Reduction and alkylation steps were performed as previously described (Görg et al. 1988). Protein separation in the second dimension was carried out in a MiniProtean III Cell (Bio-Rad). After completion of SDS-PAGE, the resulting gels were stained using ProteoSilver™ silver stain kit (Sigma-Aldrich, St. Louis, USA) according to the manufacturer's protocol. For Western blot experiments, 75 μg of pollen proteins were resolved in 2-D gels as described above. Then, proteins were electroblotted onto a PVDF membrane in a TransBlot Turbo Transfer System (Bio-Rad). Membranes were blocked overnight at 4°C in a solution containing 3% (w/v) BSA in TBS buffer (pH 7.4), and probed with primary and the corresponding secondary antibodies according to Table 1.

Images were acquired in a Pharos FX molecular imager (Bio-Rad) using the Quantity One v4.6.2 software (Bio-Rad). The reproducibility of results was confirmed by running each experiment in triplicate.

Target	Primary antibody (source)[a]	Dilution	Secondary antibody (source)	Dilution
Ole e 1	Mouse anti-olive Ole e 1 mAb (Lauzurica et al. 1988)	1:5,000	Goat anti-mouse IgG Ab, DyLight 633-conjugated (Agrisera, Vännäs, Sweden)	1:10,000
Ole e 2	Rabbit anti-olive Ole e 2 PoAb (Morales et al. 2008)	1:10,000	Donkey anti-rabbit IgG Ab, DyLight 549-conjugated (Agrisera)	1:10,000
Ole e 7	Chicken anti-olive Ole e 7 synthetic peptide PoAb	1:250	Mouse anti-chicken IgG Ab, DyLight 488-conjugated (Agrisera)	1:1,000
Ole e 9	Chicken anti-olive Ole e 9 synthetic peptide PoAb	1:5,000	Mouse anti-chicken IgG Ab, DyLight 488-conjugated (Agrisera)	1:1,000
Olive pollen allergens	Sera from olive allergic patients	1:100	Goat anti-human Ab, peroxidase-conjugated (Sigma-Aldrich)	1:10,000

Table 1. Primary and secondary antibodies and the corresponding dilutions used for 2-D Western blotting and IgE-binding experiments. Footnotes: a) mAb, monoclonal antibody; PoAb, polyclonal antibody.

A representative 2-D gel pattern of the olive pollen proteome (cv. 'Picual') containing approximately 1,400 spots is shown in Fig. 1. The global protein 2-D map was largely reproducible among replicas and the number of spots was similar to that previously reported in this cultivar (Castro et al. 2010). It was noticeable the presence of a string of prominent spots of about 20 kDa distributed along the whole pH range, forming the so-called "train". Densitometric studies indicated that the sum of these spots may represent about 15% of the total protein displayed in gels.

The distribution of Ole e 1 isoforms on 2-D polyacrylamide gels was studied using an anti-Ole e 1 antibody, namely 10H1 (Lauzurica et al. 1988). This antibody was able to recognize up to 12 different immunoreactive protein spots in the molecular weight range of 18-22 kDa (Fig. 2A). The Ole e 1 distribution pattern was identical to that previously reported (Castro et al. 2010), but a new non-glycosylated isoform was detected in the present work (Fig. 3A, spot 11). A single spot matched with a 22 kDa hyperglycosylated isoform of Ole e 1 (Villalba et al. 1993 & Castro et al. 2010). Four major and four minor spots showed an apparent molecular weight of 20 kDa and pI values between 5.1 and 8.0. They are different monoglycosylated isoforms of the allergen (Villalba et al. 1993 & Castro et al. 2010). Finally, two minor spots with pI values between 5.5 and 6.0 corresponded to two different 18.5 kDa non-glycosylated isoforms of Ole e 1 (Villalba et al. 1993 & Castro et al. 2010). Since proteins were electrophoresed under reducing conditions, we did not detect the dimer form of Ole e 1. All these immunodetected spots fitted well in their positions on the membrane with the "train of spots" visualised on 2-D gels after silver staining (Fig. 1).

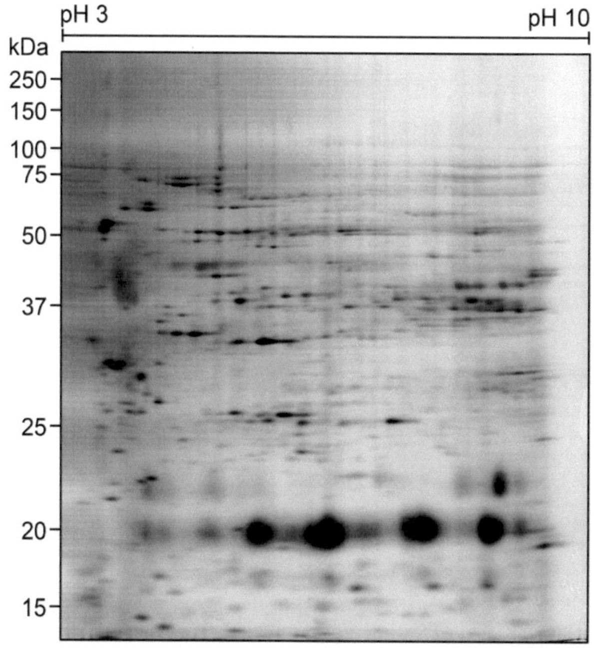

Figure 1. Representative gel of the olive pollen proteome after 2-D electrophoresis and silver staining. Approximately 75 µg of pollen total protein was loaded. Numbers at the top of the gel denote the pH gradient in the first dimension (IEF), while protein weight markers (SDS-PAGE) are shown on the left.

Using an anti-Ole e 2 polyclonal serum, we studied the number and distribution of Ole e 2 isoforms on 2-D polyacrylamide gels. Thus, two major spots of 14.3 and 13.9 kDa and a minor spot with an apparent molecular weight of 13.3 kDa were detected on 2-D blots (Fig. 2B). The three Ole e 2 isoforms are acidic and show pI values between 4.5 and 5.1.

The anti-Ole e 7 antibody revealed the presence of two different isoforms of this allergen in the olive pollen (Fig. 2C). Both proteins showed a molecular weight of approximately 10 kDa and exhibited pI values slightly acidic (6.6-6.8).

The anti-Ole e 9 antibody was able to recognize six immunoreactive protein spots of about 46 kDa and pI values between 5.8 and 6.7 (Fig. 2D). The number of spots is higher and pIs are different compared with other Ole e 9 isoforms previously described (Huecas et al. 2009). This is likely because the genetic origin of pollen samples used by Huecas et al. (2009) is different. Control reactions using the corresponding preimmune sera lacked of reactivity in all cases (results not shown).

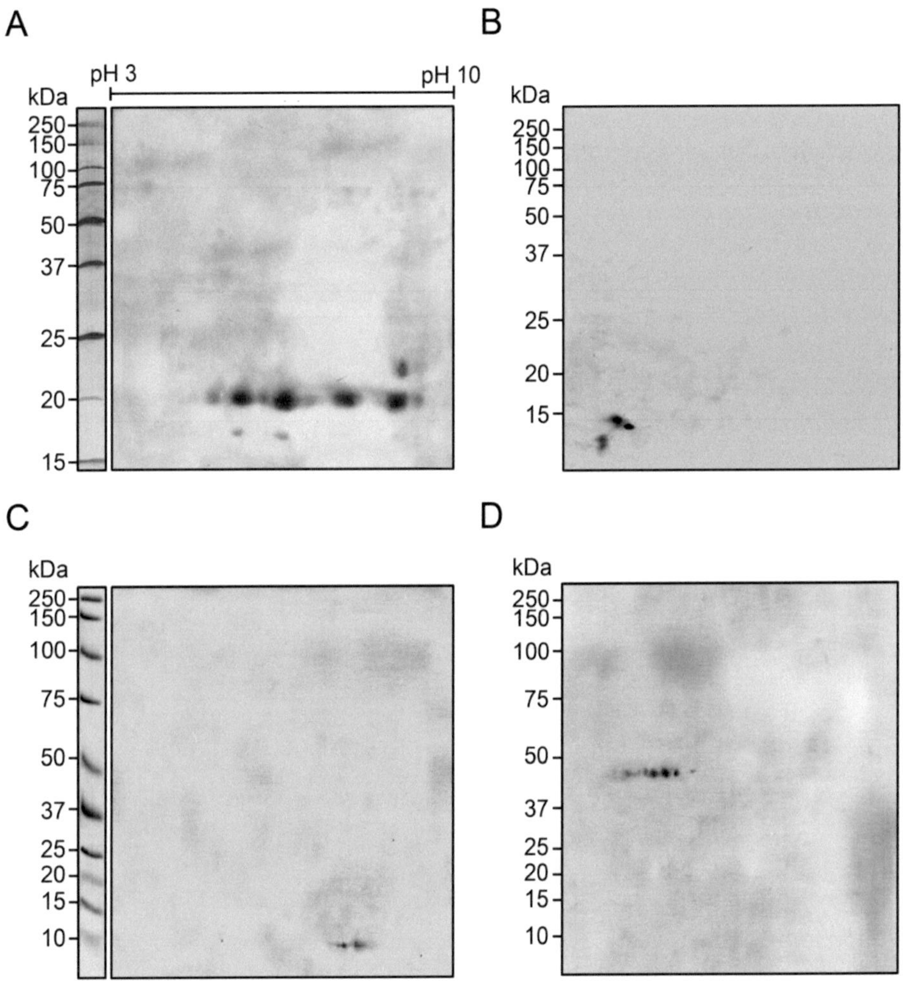

Figure 2. Detection of olive pollen allergens Ole e 1 (A), Ole e 2 (B), Ole e 7 (C) and Ole e 9 (D) on 2-D Western blot. Approximately 75 μg of pollen total protein was loaded per each gel. Numbers at the top of the gel denote the pH gradient in the first dimension (IEF), while protein weight markers are shown on the left.

3.2. Quantitation of olive pollen allergen isoforms after 2-D Western blotting

After scanning the resulting blots in a Pharos FX Plus Molecular Imager (Bio-Rad), the relative amount (%) of each allergen isoform was calculated using the Quantity One v. 4.6.2 software (Bio-Rad). Spots reactive to each antibody were defined with the help of the tool "contour" and quantitation of each spot was calculated using the "volume" parameter, defined as the total signal intensity of the pixels × area of a single pixel, inside the defined boundary drawn for each spot (Morales et al. 2012). This intensity was compared with that of the background, in a previous calibration procedure. Densitometric data of Ole e 1, Ole e 2, Ole e 7 and Ole e 9 allergen isoforms are shown in Fig. 3.

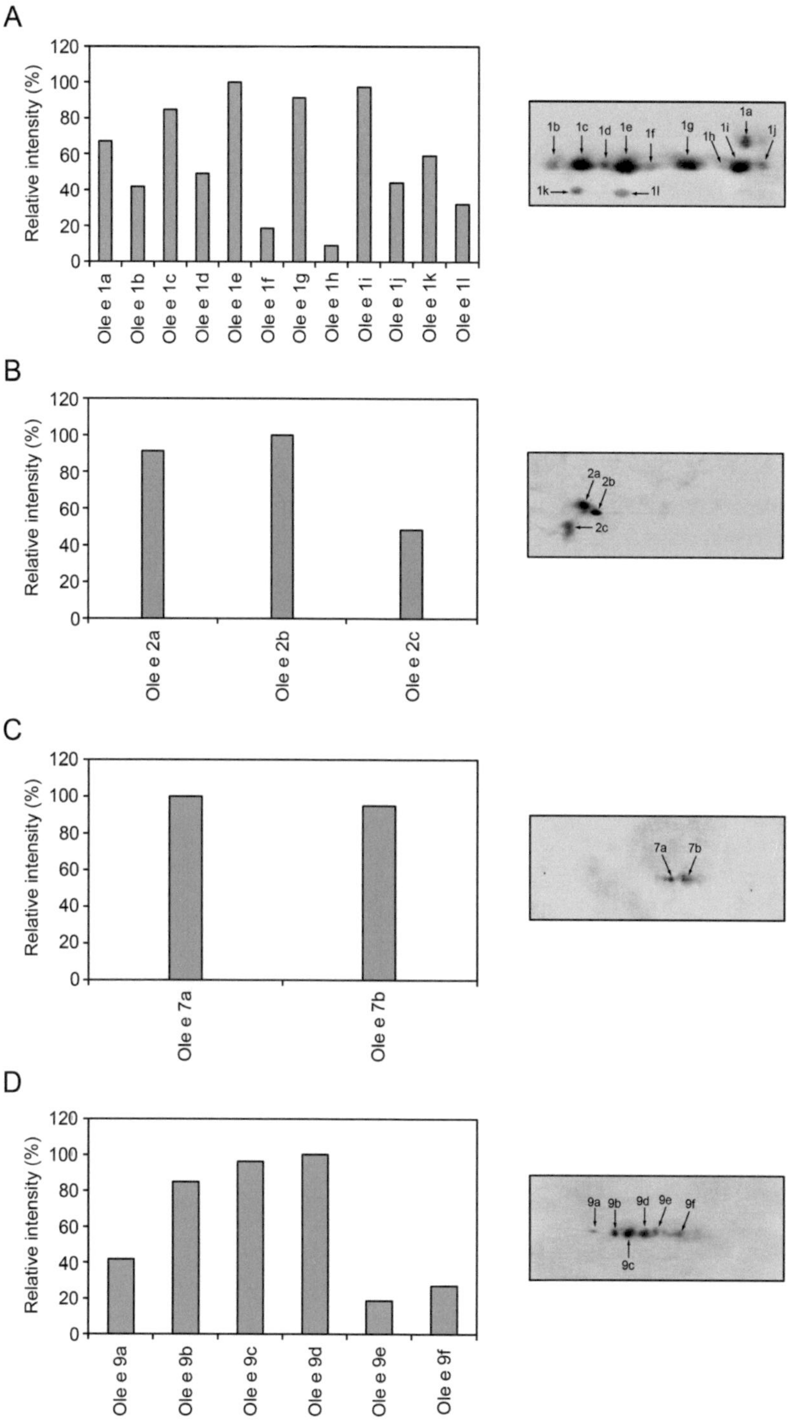

Figure 3. Quantitative analysis of Ole e 1 (A), Ole e 2 (B), Ole e 7 (C) and Ole e 9 (D) isoforms detected on 2-D blots from Fig. 2.

Ole e 1 isoforms showed the highest quantitative differences (Fig. 3A). Thus, the 12 Ole e 1 isoforms detected on 2D blots could be grouped on the basis of their intensities into 3 quantitative classes: high (>50% intensity; isoforms Ole e 1a, c, e, g and i), medium (20-50%; Ole e 1b, d, j, k and l) and low abundant (<20%; Ole e 1f and h). On the other hand, the six Ole e 9 isoforms were discriminated as high (Ole e 9a, b, c and d) or low (Ole e 9e and f) abundant (Fig. 3D). Ole e 2a and b isoforms showed similar intensities, while the amount of Ole e 2c was lower but still significant. Finally, the two Ole e 7 isoforms identified showed similar quantities.

3.3. IgE-binding analysis by 2-D Western blotting

The IgE reactivity of 'Picual' pollen proteins was assayed on 2-D blots using a pool of three olive allergic patients' sera and an anti-human IgE peroxidase-conjugated secondary antibody. Chemiluminiscent detection of IgE-binding was carried out with the Immun-Star™ WesternC™ Chemiluminescence Kit (Bio-Rad) according to the manufacturer´s instructions. Chemiluminiscent spots were imaged with a ChemiDoc XRS Molecular Imager (Bio-Rad).

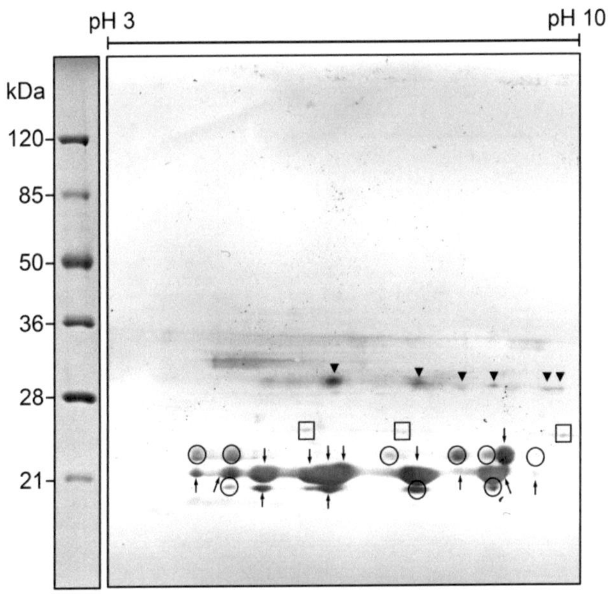

Figure 4. IgE-binding analysis by 2-D Western blotting of olive (cv. 'Picual') pollen total proteins. The blot was probed with a pool of sera from three patients allergic to olive pollen. Reactive spots were visible on the 2-D blot after detection by chemiluminiscence. Protein markers are displayed on the left.

The IgE-binding pattern is shown in Fig. 4. Incubation of the 2-D blot with patient's sera revealed up to 31 IgE-reactive spots with molecular weights ranging from 18,5 to 32 kDa. Allergic patients' IgEs recognized the 12 Ole e 1 isoforms detected by 10H1 antibody (Fig. 4, arrows). In addition, 9 new spots that might correspond to other Ole e 1 isoforms were also detected by sera (Fig. 4, circles). The remaining spots (Fig.4, squares and arrowheads) did not match with any of the Ole e 2, Ole e 7 and Ole e 9 isoforms identified previously by 2-D Western blotting (Fig. 2).

4. Conclusions

Two-dimensional Western blotting is a suitable method for olive pollen allergen isoform profiling, and might help in the standardization of protein extracts used for allergy diagnosis and immunotherapy. The 2-D electrophoresis-based immunodetection of allergens has a few advantages over classical 1-D Western-blotting, since they provide: 1) detailed information about individual isoforms of polymorphic allergens (i.e. number of isoforms, pIs and their positions on the 2-D map), and 2) relative quantitative data of each isoform. In addition, using a pool or individual sera from an allergic population, it is possible to identify which are the most reactive isoforms of a given allergen. In the present work, four allergens, namely Ole e 1, Ole e 2, Ole e 7 and Ole e 9, have been studied in a single variety (i.e. 'Picual'). These analyses should extend to other olive allergenic proteins and a higher number of cultivars. Moreover, this method can be also applied to other allergenic pollens and other type of allergies (e.g. food allergens).

Author details

Krzysztof Zienkiewicz, Estefanía García-Quirós, Juan de Dios Alché,
María Isabel Rodríguez-García and Antonio Jesús Castro
Department of Biochemistry, Cell and Molecular Biology of Plants,
Estación Experimental del Zaidín, C.S.I.C., Granada, Spain

Acknowledgement

This work was supported by the Spanish Ministry of Science and Innovation (MICINN) (ERDF-cofinanced projects AGL2008-00517, BFU2011-22779 and PIE-200840I186) and the Junta de Andalucía (ERDF-cofinanced projects P2010-CVI5767 and P2010-AGR6274). The authors thank Dr. Fernando Florido (Allergy Unit, Hospital Clínico San Cecilio, Granada, Spain) for kindly providing the sera from allergic patients. K. Zienkiewicz thanks the CSIC for providing JAEdoc grant funding.

5. References

Alché, J.D., Castro, A.J., Jiménez-López, J.C., Morales, S., Zafra, A., Hamman-Khalifa, A.M. & Rodríguez-García, M.I. (2007). Differential characteristics of olive pollen from different cultivars: biological and clinical implications. *Journal of Investigational Allergology & Clinical Immunology*, Vol. 17, Suppl 1., pp. 63-68.

Alché, J.D., Castro, A.J., Olmedilla, A., Fernández, M.C., Rodríguez, R., Villalba, M. & Rodríguez-García, M.I. (1999). The major olive pollen allergen (Ole e I) shows both gametophytic and sporophytic expression during anther development, and its synthesis and storage takes place in the RER. *Journal of Cell Science*, Vol. 112, No. 15, pp. 2501-2509.

Alché, J.D., Cismondi, I.D., Castro, A.J., Hamman Khalifa, A., & Rodríguez García, M.I. (2003). Temporal and spatial gene expression of Ole e 3 allergen in olive (*Olea europaea* L.) pollen. *Acta Biologica Cracoviensia, Series Botanica*, Vol. 45, No. 1, pp. 89-95.

Alché, J.D., Corpas, F., Rodríguez-García, M.I., & del Río, L.A. (1998). Identification and immunolocalization of superoxide dismutase isoenzymes of olive pollen. *Physiologia Plantarum*, Vol. 104, No. 4, pp. 772-776.

Alché, J.D., M'rani-Alaoui, M., Castro, A.J., & Rodríguez-García, M.I. (2004). Ole e 1, the major allergen from olive (*Olea europaea* L.) pollen, increases its expression and is released to the culture medium during in vitro germination. *Plant & Cell Physiology*, Vol. 45, No. 9, pp. 1149-1157.

Asturias, J.A., Arilla, M.C., Gómez-Bayon, N., Martínez, J., Martínez, A., & Palacios, R. (1997). Cloning and expression of the panallergen profilin and the major allergen (Ole e 1) from olive tree pollen. *Journal of Allergy & Clinical Immunology*, Vol. 100, No. 3, pp. 365-372.

Baldo, B.A. (1983). Standardization of allergens. Examination of existing procedures and the likely impact of new techniques on the quality control of extracts. *Allergy*, Vol. 38, No. 8, pp. 535–546.

Baluska, F. & Volkmann, D. (2002). Actin-driven polar growth of plant cells. *Trends in Cell Biology*, Vol. 12, No. 1, p. 14.

Barral, P., Suarez, C., Batanero, E., Alfonso, C., Alché, J. D., Rodríguez-García, M.I., Villalba, M., Rivas, G. & Rodríguez, R. (2005). An olive pollen protein with allergenic activity, Ole e 10, defines a novel family of carbohydrate-binding modules and is potentially implicated in pollen germination. *Biochemical Journal*, Vol. 390, No. 1, pp. 77-84.

Batanero, E., Crespo, J.F., Monsalve, R.I., Martín-Esteban, M., Villalba, M. & Rodríguez, R. (1999). IgE-binding and histamine-release capabilities of the main carbohydrate component isolated from the major allergen of olive tree pollen, Ole e 1. *Journal of Allergy & Clinical Immunology*, Vol. 103, No. 1, pp. 147-153.

Batanero, E., Ledesma, A., Villalba, M., & Rodríguez, R. (1997). Purification, amino acid sequence and immunological characterization of Ole e 6, a cysteine-enriched allergen from olive tree pollen. *FEBS Letters*, Vol. 410, No. 2-3, pp. 293-296.

Batanero, E., Villalba, M., Ledesma, A., Puente, X.S., & Rodríguez, R. (1996a). Ole e 3, an olive-tree allergen, belongs to a widespread family of pollen proteins. *European Journal of Biochemistry*, Vol. 241, No. 3, pp. 772-778.

Batanero, E., Villalba, M., Monsalve, R.I., & Rodríguez R. (1996b). Cross-reactivity between the major allergen from olive pollen and unrelated glycoproteins: evidence of an epitope in the glycan moiety of the allergen. *Journal of Allergy & Clinical Immunology*, Vol.97, No.6, pp. 1264-1271.

Batanero, E., Villalba, M. & Rodríguez, R. (1994). Glycosylation site of the major allergens from olive tree pollen. Allergenic implications of the carbohydrate moiety. *Molecular Immunology*, Vol. 31, No. 1, pp. 31-37.

Boluda, L., Alonso, C., & Fernández-Caldas, E. (1998). Purification, characterization, and partial sequencing of two new allergens of *Olea europaea*. *Journal of Allergy & Clinical Immunology*, Vol. 101, No. 2, pp. 210-216.

Bosch, M., Cheung, A.Y. & Hepler, P.K. (2005). Pectin methylesterase, a regulator of pollen tube growth. *Plant Physiology*, Vol. 138, pp. 1334–1346.

Butteroni, C., Afferni, C., Barletta, B., Iacovacci, P., Corinti, S., Brunetto, B., Tinghino, R., Ariano, R., Panzani, R.C., Pini. C., & Di Felice, G. (2005). Cloning and Expression of the *Olea europaea* allergen Ole e 5, the pollen Cu/Zn superoxide dismutase. *International Archives of Allergy & Immunology*, Vol. 137, No. 1, pp. 9-17.

Castro, A.J., Alché, J.D., Cuevas, J., Romero, P.J., Alché, V., & Rodríguez-García, M.I. (2003). Pollen from different olive tree cultivars contains varying amounts of the major allergen Ole e 1. *International Archives of Allergy & Immunology*, Vol. 131, No. 3, pp. 164-173.

Castro, A.J., Bednarczyk, A., Schaeffer-Reiss, C., Rodríguez-García, M., Van Dorsselaer, A., & Alché, J.D. (2010) Screening of Ole e 1 polymorphism among olive cultivars by peptide mapping and N-glycopeptide analysis. *Proteomics*, Vol. 10, No. 5, pp. 953-962.

Díaz-Perales, A., Lombardero, M., Sánchez-Monge, R., García-Selles, F.J., Pernas, M., Fernández-Rivas, M., Barber, D., & Salcedo, G. (2000). Lipid-transfer proteins as potential plant panallergens: cross-reactivity among proteins of *Artemisia* pollen, Castaneae nut and Rosaceae fruits, with different IgE-binding capacities. *Clinical & Experimental Allergy*, Vol. 30, No. 10, pp. 1403-1410.

Engel, E., Richter, K., Obermeyer, G., Briza, P., Kungl, A. J., Simon, B., Auer, M., Ebner, C., Rheinberger, H. J., Breitenbach, M., & Ferreira, F. (1997) Immunological and biological properties of Bet v 4, a novel birch pollen allergen with two EF-hand calcium-binding domains. *Journal of Biological Chemistry*, Vol. 272, No. 45, pp. 28630–28637.

Esteve, C., Montealegre, C., Marina, M.L., & García, M.C. (2012). Analysis of olive allergens. *Talanta*, Vol. 92, pp. 1-14.

González, E.M., Villalba, M., Lombardero, M., Aalbers, M., van Ree, R., & Rodríguez, R. (2002). Influence of the 3D-conformation, glycan component and microheterogeneity on the epitope structure of Ole e 1, the major olive allergen. Use of recombinant isoforms and specific monoclonal antibodies as immunological tools. *Molecular Immunology*, Vol. 39, No. 1-2, pp. 93-101.

Görg, A., Postel, W., & Günther, S. (1988). Two-dimensional electrophoresis. The current state of two-dimensional electrophoresis with immobilized pH gradients. *Electrophoresis*, Vol. 9, No. 9, pp. 531–546.

Hamman Khalifa A, Castro, A.J., Rodríguez García, M.I., & Alché, J.D (2008). Olive cultivar origin is a major cause of polymorphism for Ole e 1 pollen allergen. *BMC Plant Biology*, Vol. 8, pp. 10.

Hayek, B., Vangelista, L., Pastore, A., Sperr, W. R., Valent, P., Vrtala, S., Niederberger, V., Twardosz, A., Kraft, D., & Valenta, R. (1998). Molecular and immunologic characterization of a highly cross-reactive two EF-hand calcium-binding alder pollen allergen, Aln g 4: structural basis for calcium-modulated IgE recognition. *Journal of Immunology*, Vol. 161, No. 12, pp. 7031– 7039.

Huecas, S., Villalba, M., & Rodríguez, R. (2001). Ole e 9, a major olive pollen allergen is a 1,3-beta-glucanase. Isolation, characterization, amino acid sequence, and tissue specificity. *Journal of Biological Chemistry*, Vol. 276, No. 30, pp. 27959-27966.

Jiang, L., Yang, S.L., Xie, L.F., Puah, C.S., Zhang, X.Q., Yang, W.C., Sundaresan, V. & Ye, D.. (2005). VANGUARD1 encodes a pectin methylesterase that enhances pollen tube growth in the *Arabidopsis* style and transmitting tract. *The Plant Cell*, Vol. 17, pp. 584–596.

Jiménez-López, J.C., Morales, S., Castro, A.J., Volkmann, D., Rodríguez-García, M.I. & Alché, J.D. (2012). Characterization of profilin polymorphism in pollen with a focus on multifunctionality. *PLoS One*, Vol. 7, No. 2, p. e30878.

Karlsson, R. & Lindberg, U. (2007). Profilin, an essential control element for actin polymerization. In *Actin monomer-binding proteins*, Lappalainen P. (ed.), Landes Bioscience, Georgetown.

Lauzurica, P., Gurbindo, C., Maruri, N., Galocha, B., Díaz, R., González, J., García, R. & Lahoz, C. (1988). Olive (*Olea europaea*) pollen allergens. I. Immunochemical characterization by immunoblotting, CRIE and immunodetection by a monoclonal antibody. *Molecular Immunology*, Vol. 25, pp. 329-335.

Ledesma, A., Rodríguez, R., & Villalba, M. (1998a). Olive-pollen profilin. Molecular and immunologic properties. *Allergy* Vol. 53, No. 5, pp. 520-526.

Ledesma, A., Villalba, M., & Rodríguez, R. (2000). Cloning, expression and characterization of a novel four EF-hand Ca($^{2+}$)-binding protein from olive pollen with allergenic activity. *FEBS Letters*, Vol. 466, No. 1, pp. 192-196.

Ledesma, A., Villalba, M., Batanero, E., & Rodríguez, R. (1998b). Molecular cloning and expression of active Ole e 3, a major allergen from olive-tree pollen and member of a novel family of Ca^{2+}-binding proteins (polcalcins) involved in allergy. *European Journal of Biochemistry*, Vol. 258, No. 2, pp. 454-459.

Ledesma, A., Villalba, M., Vivanco, F., & Rodríguez, R. (2002). Olive pollen allergen Ole e 8: identification in mature pollen and presence of Ole e 8-like proteins in different pollens. *Allergy*, Vol. 57, No. 1, pp. 40-43.

Lombardero, M., Quirce, S., Duffort, O., Barber, D., Carpizo, J., Chamorro, M.J., Lezaun, A., & Carreira, J. (1992). Monoclonal antibodies against *Olea europaea* major allergen: allergenic activity of affinity-purified allergen and depleted extract and development of a radioimmunoassay for the quantitation of the allergen. *Journal of Allergy & Clinical Immunology*, Vol. 89, pp. 884-894.

Martínez, A., Asturias, J.A., Monteseirín, J., Moreno, V., García-Cubillana, A., Hernández, M., de la Calle, A., Sánchez-Hernández, C., Pérez-Formoso, J.L., & Conde, J. (2002). The allergenic relevance of profilin (Ole e 2) from *Olea europaea* pollen. *Allergy*, Vol. 57, Suppl. 71, pp. 17-23.

Morales, S., Castro, A.J., Jiménez-López, J.C., Florido, F., Rodríguez-García, M.I., & Alché J.D. (2012). A novel multiplex method for the simultaneous detection and relative quantification of pollen allergens. *Electrophoresis*, Vol. 33, DOI 10.1002/elps.201100667.

Morales, S., Jiménez-López, J.C., Castro, A.J., Rodríguez-García, M.I., & Alché, J.D. (2008). Olive pollen profilin (Ole e 2 allergen) co-localizes with highly active areas of the actin cytoskeleton and is released to the culture medium during in vitro pollen germination. *Journal of Microscopy-Oxford*, Vol. 231, No. 2, pp. 332-341.

Movérare, R., Westritschnig, K., Svensson, M., Hayek, B., Bende, M., Pauli, G., Sorva, R., Haahtela, T., Valenta, R., & Elfman, L. (2002). Different IgE reactivity profiles in birch pollen-sensitive patients from six European populations revealed by recombinant allergens: an imprint of local sensitization. *International Archives of Allergy & Immunology*, Vol. 128, No. 4, pp. 325-335.

Quiralte, J., Palacios, L., Rodríguez, R., Cardaba, B., Arias de Saavedra, J.M., Villalba, M., Florido, J.F,. & Lahoz, C. (2007). Modelling diseases: the allergens of *Olea europaea* pollen. *Journal of Investigational Allergology & Clinical Immunology*, Vol. 17, Suppl. 1, pp. 24-30.

Rodríguez, R., Villalba, M., Batanero, E., González, E.M., Monsalve, R.I., Huecas, S., Tejera, M.L., & Ledesma, A. (2002). Allergenic diversity of the olive pollen. *Allergy*, Vol. 57, Suppl. 71, pp. 6-16.

Salamanca, G., Rodríguez, R., Quiralte, J., Moreno, C., Pascual, C.Y., Barber, D., & Villalba, M. (2010). Pectin methylesterases of pollen tissue, a major allergen in olive tree. *FEBS Journal*, Vol. 277, No. 13, pp. 2729-2739.

Santos, A., & Van Ree, R. (2011). Profilins: mimickers of allergy or relevant allergens? *International Archives of Allergy & Immunology*, Vol.155, No. 3, pp. 191-204.

Tejera, M.L., Villalba, M., Batanero, E., & Rodríguez, R. (1999). Identification, isolation, and characterization of Ole e 7, a new allergen of olive tree pollen. *The Journal of Allergy & Clinical Immunology*, Vol. 104, No. 4, pp. 797-802.

Treviño, M.A., Palomares, O., Castrillo, I., Villalba, M., Rodríguez, R., Rico, M., Santoro, J., & Bruix, M. (2008). Solution structure of the C-terminal domain of Ole e 9, a major allergen of olive pollen. *Protein Science*, Vol. 17, No. 2, pp. 371-376.

Twardosz, A., Hayek, B., Seiberler, S., Vangelista, L., Elfman, L., Grönlund, H., Kraft, D., & Valenta, R. (1997). Molecular characterization, expression in *Escherichia coli*, and epitope analysis of a two EF-hand calcium-binding birch pollen allergen, Bet v 4. *Biochemical & Biophysical Research Communications*, Vol. 239, No. 1, pp. 197-204.

Valenta, R., Duchene, M., Ebner, C., Valent, P., Sillaber, C., Deviller, P., Ferreira, F., Tejkl, M., Edelmann, H., Kraft, D., & Scheiner, O. (1992). Profilins constitute a novel family of functional plant pan-allergens. *The Journal of Experimental Medicine*, Vol. 175, No. 2, pp. 377-385.

Van Ree, R. (1997). Analytic aspects of the standardization of allergenic extracts. *Allergy*, Vol. 52, No. 8, pp. 795-805.

Van Ree, R. (2007). Indoor allergens: relevance of major allergen measurements and standardization. *The Journal of Allergy and Clinical Immunology*, Vol. 119, No. 2, pp. 270-277.

Villalba, M., Batanero, E., Lopez-Otín, C., Sánchez, L.M., Monsalve, R.I., González de la Peña, M.A., Lahoz, C., & Rodríguez, R. (1993). The amino acid sequence of Ole e I, the major allergen from olive tree (*Olea europaea*) pollen. *European Journal of Biochemistry*, Vol. 216, No. 3, pp. 863-869.

Villalba, M., Batanero, E., Monsalve, R.I., González de la Peña, M.A. Lahoz, C., & Rodríguez, R. (1994). Cloning and expression of Ole e I, the major allergen from olive tree pollen. Polymorphism analysis and tissue specificity. *Journal of Biological Chemistry*, Vol. 269, No. 21, pp. 15217-15222.

Chapter 4

Involvement of Climatic Factors in the Allergen Expression in Olive Pollen

Sonia Morales, Antonio Jesús Castro,
María Isabel Rodríguez-García and Juan de Dios Alché

Additional information is available at the end of the chapter

http://dx.doi.org/10.5772/50077

1. Introduction

Olive allergen concentrations in the pollen grain are critical in allergic response of atopic patients. Existing evidence shows that climatic factors can influence pollen allergen content. To date, the influences of temperature and precipitations over the content of birch and olive pollens in their respective major allergens have been analyzed. Bet v 1, the major allergen of birch pollen, increased its expression (Buters et al. 2008) and presented a higher allergenicity (Ahlholm et al. 1998) while temperatures were elevated. Differently, the content in the major olive pollen allergen Ole e 1 showed no apparent correlation with either temperatures or precipitations (Fernández Caldas et al. 2007). However, a positive correlation between total allergenicity and rainfall occurring in winter months was found. This correlation was not analyzed independently for each pollen allergen.

Our aim was to extend the observations carried out in olive pollen, by analyzing the effects of climate parameters over the expression of four olive pollen allergens. Using a recently developed multiplex western blotting system for the assessment of allergenic molecules (Morales et al. 2012), we have simultaneously detected and quantified two major (Ole e 1 and Ole e 9) and two minor allergens (Ole e 2 and Ole e 5) in the pollen extracts from seven olive cultivars collected along 4-7 consecutive years. The considered climatic variables included temperature, precipitation, number of rain days and humidity. Data were provided by the Spanish network for the temporal observation of ecosystems (REDOTE). Correlations between the allergen contents (both individually and all inclusive) and climate variables were studied by applying Spearman correlation tests. Results showed significant variations in the expression of the four allergens in the seven cultivars throughout the years of the analysis. All these positive correlations corresponded exactly to the period of time starting the winter prior to each flowering period to the end of period (this is, December from the previous year to June).

These results are discussed as regard to their putative incidence in the development of symptoms by patients, the requirements for medical assistance and the rates of admission into clinical centres and hospitals. Agronomical implications in olive sexual reproduction, including fruit setting and fruit production, are also discussed.

2. Materials and methods

2.1. Pollen samples

Olea europaea L. pollen samples were obtained during May and June of 2000-2007 from cultivated trees of the cultivars: 'Arbequina', 'Blanqueta', 'Hojiblanca', 'Manzanilla de Sevilla', 'Picual', 'Verdial de Huévar' and 'Verdial de Vélez' situated at the IFAPA center "Alameda del Obispo" (Andalusian Regional Government, Córdoba, Spain). Pollen samples were collected from numerous branches of at least two trees of each cultivar by shaking flowering shoots inside paper bags. Prior to its storage in liquid nitrogen, the harvested pollen was sieved through a 150 μm mesh in order to eliminate fallen corollas, anthers and other rests. After light microscopy observation, foreign-species pollen was estimated to be <0.1% and other plant parts <0.5% for all the cultivars used.

2.2. Preparation of crude protein extracts and SDS-PAGE

Crude protein extracts were obtained by stirring 1 g of pollen for each cultivar in 10 ml extraction buffer (0.01 M ammonium bicarbonate, pH 8.0, and 2 mM phenylmethylsulfonyl fluoride) for 8 h at 4°C. After centrifugation (2 x 30 minutes at 14,000 rpm at 4°C), the supernatants were filtered through a 0.2 μm filter, and stored in aliquots at –20°C. Protein concentration in the different samples was measured using the Bio-Rad reagent (Bio-Rad, Hercules, CA, USA) and bovine serum albumin (BSA) as standard.

Proteins (30 μg per lane) and Mw1 (New England BioLabs, Ipswich, MA, USA) and Mw2 standards (MBI Fermentas, Vilnius, Lithuania) were separated by sodium dodecyl sulfate-polyacrylamide gel electrophoresis (SDS-PAGE) in 15% gels in a MiniProtean II system (Bio-Rad). The resulting gels were stained with silver nitrate (Rabilloud et al., 1994).

2.3. Immunoblotting

Gels obtained as described above were transferred onto BioTrace® polyvinylidene difluoride (PVDF) membranes (Pall BioSupport, Port Washington, NY, USA) at 100 V for 1.5 hours using a Mini Trans-Blot Electrophoretic Transfer Cell (Bio-Rad). Prior to the treatment with antibodies, the membranes were blocked with TBST buffer (Tris buffered saline: TBS + 0.3% v/v Tween 20) + 10% w/v dried skimmed milk. For membrane probing, a recently developed multiplex Western blotting system for the assessment of allergenic molecules (Morales et al. 2012) has been used. Briefly, the simultaneous detection of four olive pollen allergens (Ole e 1, Ole e 2, Ole e 5 and Ole e 9) on a single blot using a monoclonal antibody from mouse and three polyclonal antibodies raised in rabbit is carried out. We utilized unconjugated Fab antibody fragments for blocking rabbit primary antibodies, and fluorescence-based detection. These changes allowed an accurate and reliable comparative quantitation of these allergens among pollen protein samples.

2.4. Absolute and relative quantitation of allergens

Imaging was carried out with a Pharos FX Plus Molecular Imager (Bio-Rad) using the Quantity One v4.6.2 software (Bio-Rad). The intensity of each fluorescent band was calculated using the quantitation tools of the Quantity One v4.6.2 software.

2.5. Climate parameters

Climate parameters were obtained from the weather tracking station situated at Córdoba airport (Spain) during the years 2000 to 2007. Information was extracted from the Spanish long term ecological research network (REDOTE).

2.6. Statistical analysis

Continuous variables were subjected to a study of normality distribution by using the Kolmorov-Smirnov test. Associations between continuous variables (non-normal distribution) were described by analysis of bivariate Spearman correlation (two-tailed). Significant correlation was considered $P<0.05$.

3. Results

3.1. Multiplex determination of year-to-year allergen expression in seven olive cultivars

Figure 1A shows the protein profiles of the extracts analyzed after SDS-PAGE and silver staining. The different panels correspond to the cultivars analyzed between the years 2000 and 2007. Bands were observed in the range of 15 to 75 kDa. Clear quantitative differences were distinguished, from which the most conspicuous were those in the bands of 20 kDa and 18.4 kDa among de different years, with the exception of cultivars 'Arbequina', 'Verdial de Huévar' and 'Hojiblanca', in which the Ole e 1 bands were not well identified after silver staining. The remaining allergens studied were not identified after silver staining.

Allergenic profiles were assessed by multiplex immunotransference (Figure 1B). The cultivars 'Arbequina' and 'Hojiblanca' displayed two Ole e 1 forms (20 kDa and 18.4 kDa) in contrast with the remaining cultivars, were the three major forms of Ole e 1 (22 kDa, 20 kDa and 18.4 kDa) were distinguished. Differences in the expression of this allergen depending on the year of pollen collection can be easily noticed.

Ole e 2 was visualized in all cultivars in the form of two bands with sizes of 15.1 kDa and 14 kDa, with the exception of the 'Verdial de Vélez' cultivar, in which only the 15.1 kDa band was present. As described for Ole e 1, the presence of noticeable differences in the expression of the Ole e 2 allergen, depending the year of pollen collection can be observed in the corresponding multiplex immunoblots.

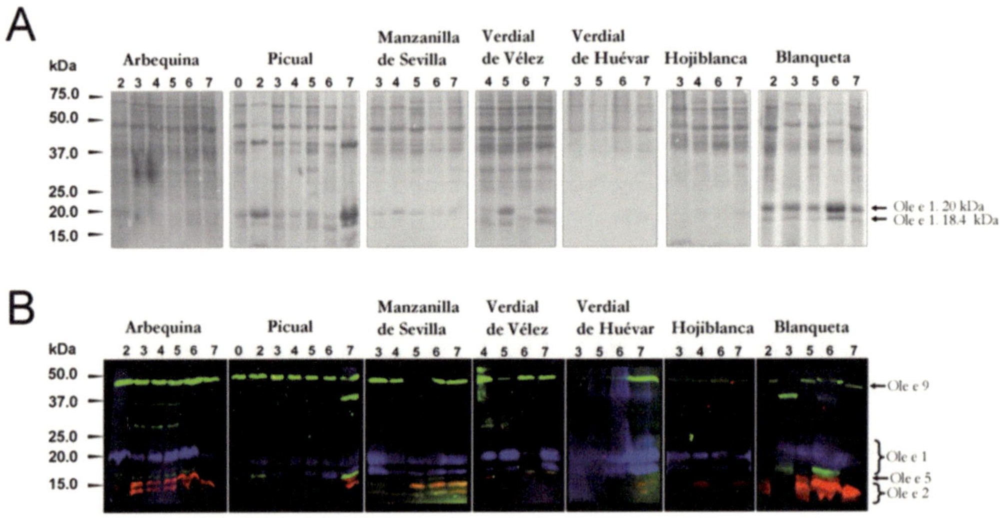

Figure 1. A) Silver staining of total protein extracts obtained from pollen corresponding to the seven cultivars analyzed trhoughout the different years. B) Multiplex detection of the allergens Ole e 1, Ole e 2, Ole e 5 and Ole e 9 in the same extracts described in panel A. Thirty micrograms of total protein were loaded in each lane. Lane numbers (0-7) correspond to the years analyzed (2000-2007). Molecular weight standards are displayed on the left.

Ole e 5 allergen can be observed in the cultivars analyzed. However, only a weak signal was detected in the cultivars 'Hojiblanca' and 'Verdial de Huévar'. Year-to-year differences in the expression of this allergen are clearly observed in 'Picual' and 'Blanqueta' cultivars.

Finally, Ole e 9 was expressed in all cultivars analyzed. Year-to-year differences in their expression are observed as well, with the sharpest differences in the cultivars 'Blanqueta' and 'Manzanilla de Sevilla'.

3.2. Involvement of climatic factors in the expression of Ole e 1 allergen

Correlation between the data corresponding to the major climatic factors and the expression of the allergens Ole e 1, Ole e 2, Ole e 5 y Ole e 9 was individually assessed for each cultivar by means of Spearman correlation analyses. The analysis of the correlation between the levels of the Ole e 1 and these climatic parameters is shown in Table 1. The presence of a statistically significant positive correlation between the expression of the different Ole e 1 forms (either individually or their added values) and the accumulated yearly average temperatures (the addition of the monthly average temperatures during those months prior to the blooming period -July of the prior year to June of the current year-) was determined for the cultivar 'Blanqueta'. Total levels of the Ole e 1 allergen correlated positively with the monthly average temperatures during the winter period (for the cultivar 'Verdial de Huévar') or the spring period (cultivars 'Blanqueta', 'Hojiblanca').

Cultivar	Climatic factor		Ole e 1 22 kDa	Ole e 1 20 kDa	Ole e 1 18.4 kDa	All Ole e 1 bands
Arbequina	Yearly AT accumulated (°C)	R	-----		.65	
		P			.156	
Blanqueta	Yearly AT accumulated (°C)	R	.9*	1**		.9*
		P	.037	<0.001		.037
	AT April (°C)	R		.9*		
		P		.037		
	AT May (°C)	R		.9*		
		P		.037		
	mT May (°C)	R	.9*	1**		0.9*
		P	.037	<0.001		.037
Hojiblanca	AT March (°C)	R	-----		1**	1**
		P			<0.001	<0.001
	mT March (°C)	R	-----		1**	1**
		P			<0.001	<0.001
	Accumulated precipitation winter (January-March) (mm)	R	-----	1**		
		P		<0.001		
	precipitation February (mm)	R	-----	1**		
		P		<0.001		
Picual	AT April (°C)	R			.643	
		P			.119	
	mT April (°C)	R	-----		.829*	
		P			.021	
	MT April (°C)	R	-----		.757*	
		P			.049	
Verdial de Vélez	No. days of rain in August	R	1**		1**	1**
		P	<0.001		<0.001	<0.001
Verdial de Huévar	AT February (°C)	R		1**	1**	1**
		P		<0.001	<0.001	<0.001
	Accumulated precipitation (January-May) (mm)	R		1**	1**	1**
		P		<0.001	<0.001	<0.001
	No. days of rain in February	R	.949	.949	.949	.949
		P	.05	.05	.05	.05
	No. days of rain in April	R	1**			
		P	<0.001			
	Accumulated mRH (January-May) (%)	R		1**	1**	1**
		P		<0.001	<0.001	<0.001
	mRH January (%)	R		1**	1**	1**
		P		<0.001	<0.001	<0.001

Cultivar	Climatic factor		Ole e 1 22 kDa	Ole e 1 20 kDa	Ole e 1 18.4 kDa	All Ole e 1 bands
	mRH February (%)	R	1**			
		P	<0.001			
	mRH April (%)	R		1**	1**	1**
		P		<0.001	<0.001	<0.001
	mRH May (%)	R		1**	1**	1**
		P		<0.001	<0.001	<0.001
Manzanilla de Sevilla	AT March (°C)	R			.8	
		P			.104	
	AT March (°C)	R			.7	
		P			.108	
	mT March (°C)	R		.9*		
		P		.037		
	MT May (°C)	R		.9*		
		P		.037		
	Accumulated yearly precipitation (mm)	R	.9*	1**		0.9*
		P	.037	.001		.037
	precipitation July (mm)	R		.894		.894
		P		.04		.04
	precipitation September (mm)	R	1**			
		P	<0.001			
	precipitation November (mm)	R	.9*	.9*		.9*
		P	.03	.037		.037
	precipitation April (mm)	R		.9*		.9*
		P		.037		.037
	No. days of rain in January	R		.9*		.9*
		P		.037		.037
	No. days of rain in April	R		.9*		.9*
		P		.037		.037
	Accumulated yearly mRH (%)	R	1**			
		P	<0.001			
	mRH December (%)	R	.9*			
		P	.037			
	mRH February (%)	R		.9*		.9*
		P		.037		.037

AT: average temperature. mT: minimum temperature. MT: maximum temperature. mRH: monthly relative humidity

Table 1. Analysis of bivariate Spearman correlation (two-tailed) between the expression of the different Ole e 1 forms both individually and jointly (CNT*mm^2) and different climatic factors. R: Spearman correlation coefficient. * Statistically significant correlation $P<0.05$; ** $P<0.01$.

Moreover, statistically significant positive correlations were observed between Ole e 1 expression and minimum temperatures (cultivars 'Blanqueta', 'Hojiblanca', 'Picual' and 'Manzanilla de Sevilla') or maximum temperatures (cultivars 'Picual' and 'Manzanilla de Sevilla') during the spring period.

Total expression of Ole e 1 correlated positively with the added monthly precipitation occurred during the winter and spring period (cultivars 'Hojiblanca' and 'Verdial de Huévar'), as well as with the total precipitation occurred during the months prior to flowering (cultivar 'Manzanilla de Sevilla'). Positive correlations are also observed between total levels of Ole e 1 allergen and precipitation, number of days of rain, and the monthly average of relative humidity during the months prior to the blooming season.

3.3. Involvement of climatic factors in the expression of Ole e 2 allergen

Table 2 displays the observed correlations between Ole e 2 and different climatic factors.

Cultivar	Climatic factor		Ole e 2 15.1 kDa	Ole e 2 14 kDa	All Ole e 2 bands
Arbequina	AT June (°C)	R	.886*		.886*
		P	.019		.019
	MT June (°C)	R	.886*		.886*
		P	.019		.019
	Accumulated precipitation winter (January-March) (mm)	R		.943**	
		P		.005	
	precipitation February (mm)	R		.943**	
		P		.005	
Hojiblanca	AT February (°C)	R	1**		
		P	<0.001		
	mT April (°C)	R			.829*
		P			.021
	MT April (°C)	R			.757*
		P			.049
	Accumulated mRH (January-May) (%)	R	1**		
		P	<0.001		
	mRH January (%)	R	1**		
		P	<0.001		
	mRH May (%)	R	1**		
		P	<0.001		
Verdial de Vélez	mRH December (%)	R			1**
		P			<0.001
Verdial de Huévar	AT January (°C)	R		1**	
		P		<0.001	
	precipitation June (mm)	R		.775*	
		P		.041	

	Accumulated No. of raining days (January-May)	R		1**	
		P		<0.001	
	No. days of rain in February	R	.949	.949	.949
		P	.05	.05	.05
	No. days of rain in April	R	1**		1**
		P	<0.001		<0.001
	Accumulated mRH (January-May) (%)	R		1**	
		P		<0.001	
	mRH February (%)	R	1**		1**
		P	<0.001		<0.001
	mRH April (%)	R	1**		
		P	<0.001		
	mRH May (%)	R	1**		
		P	<0.001		
Manzanilla de Sevilla	precipitation June (mm)	R	.949*	.949*	.949*
		P	.014	.014	.014
	No. days of rain in June	R	.872	.872	.872
		P	.05	.05	.05

Table 2. Analysis of bivariate Spearman correlation (two-tailed) between the expression of the different Ole e 2 forms both individually and jointly (CNT*mm^2) and different climatic factors. R: Spearman correlation coefficient. * Statistically significant correlation P<0.05; ** P<0.01. AT: average temperature. mT: minimum temperature. MT: maximum temperature. mRH: monthly relative humidity.

The expression levels of the bands corresponding to the Ole e 2 allergen (Table 2) and/or their addition, correlated positively with the average temperatures for particular months during the winter period (cultivars 'Hojiblanca' and 'Verdial de Huévar') or spring (cultivar 'Arbequina'). Statistically significant correlations were also observed between the expression of Ole e 2 and the maximum/minimum temperatures over the months corresponding to the spring (cultivars 'Arbequina' and 'Hojiblanca').

The expression of one of the Ole e 2 form is positively correlated to the accumulated monthly precipitation occurred during the winter months for the cultivar 'Arbequina', as well as to the precipitation occurred in particular months during the winter and spring (cultivars 'Arbequina', 'Verdial de Huévar' and 'Manzanilla de Sevilla'). The Ole e 2 form with the higher molecular weight (15.1 kDa) also presented correlation to the accumulated monthly relative humidity during the months of winter and spring (cultivars 'Hojiblanca' and 'Verdial de Huévar'). Similarly, positive correlation was detected between the total levels of Ole e 2 and the total number of days of rain over the winter and spring months (cultivar 'Verdial de Huévar').

3.4. Involvement of the climatic factors in the expression of Ole e 5 allergen

As respects to Ole e 5 allergen (Table 3), the presence of a statistically significant positive correlation was determined between the minimum temperature during May, and the precipitation observed during February in the 'Blanqueta' cultivar. In the cultivar 'Verdial de Vélez', Ole e 5 correlated to the number of days of rain and the relative humidity over the months of February and April.

Cultivar	Climatic factor		Ole e 5
Blanqueta	mT May (°C)	R	.9*
		P	.0187
	precipitation February (mm)	R	.9 *
		P	.0037
Verdial de Vélez	No. days of rain in February	R	1**
		P	<0.001
	No. days of rain in April	R	1**
		P	<0.001
	mRH February (%)	R	1**
		P	<0.001
	mRH April (%)	R	1**
		P	<0.001

Table 3. Analysis of bivariate Spearman correlation (two-tailed) between the expression of Ole e 5 (CNT*mm^2) and different climatic factors. R: Spearman correlation coefficient. *Statistically significant correlation $P<0.05$; ** $P<0.01$. AT: average temperature. mT: minimum temperature. MT: maximum temperature. mRH: monthly relative humidity.

3.5. Involvement of climatic factors in the expression of Ole e 9 allergen

As regard to the Ole e 9 allergen, its expression correlated positively (Table 4) with the average temperatures during the months of January (cultivars 'Arbequina', and 'Verdial de Huévar') and March ('Hojiblanca'). In the same way, a correlation was demonstrated between Ole e 9 expression and the number of days of rain during March in the cultivars 'Arbequina' and 'Verdial de Vélez'. The average relative humidity also showed a statistically relevant correlation during the months of winter, for the cultivar 'Picual', and specifically for January in the cultivar 'Verdial de Huévar'. In addition, and for this last cultivar 'Verdial de Huévar', the relative humidity presents a positive correlation during the spring months of April and May.

3.6. Several examples of data distributions

We describe next several examples of data distributions corresponding to climatic factors showing a statistically significant correlation with the expression level of the different allergens. Charts represent the allergen levels (represented as band intensities) plotted against climatic factors like temperature (Figure 2), precipitation, relative humidity and number of days of rain (Figure 3). A reference line showing a theoretical absolute linear correlation between the variables was added to the figures.

Cultivar	Climatic factor		Ole e 9
Arbequina	AT January (°C)	R	.829*
		P	.042
	No of days of rain in March	R	.088*
		P	.02
Hojiblanca	AT March (°C)	R	1**
		P	<0.001
	mT March (°C)	R	1**
		P	<0.001
Picual	mRH December (%)	R	.857*
		P	.014
Verdial de Vélez	No. days of rain in March	R	.949
		P	.05
Verdial de Huévar	AT January (°C)	R	1**
		P	<0.001
	No. days of rain in February	R	.949
		P	.05
	mRH January (%)	R	1**
		P	<0.001
	mRH April (%)	R	1**
		P	<0.001
	mRH May (%)	R	1**
		P	<0.001

Table 4. Analysis of bivariate Spearman correlation (two-tailed) between the expression of Ole e 9 (CNT*mm²) and different climatic factors. R: Spearman correlation coefficient. *Statistically significant correlation P<0.05; ** P<0.01. AT: average temperature. mT: minimum temperature. MT: maximum temperature. mRH: monthly relative humidity.

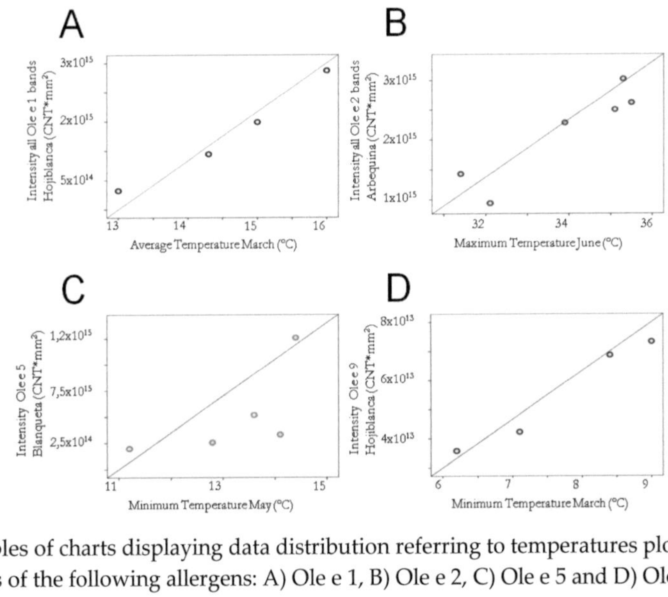

Figure 2. Examples of charts displaying data distribution referring to temperatures plotted against the expression levels of the following allergens: A) Ole e 1, B) Ole e 2, C) Ole e 5 and D) Ole e 9.

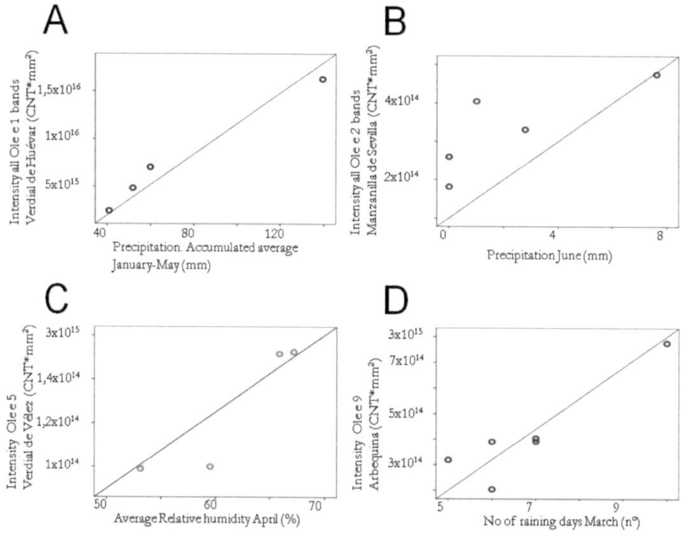

Figure 3. Examples of charts displaying data distribution referring to precipitation, relative humidity and number of days of rain plotted against the expression levels of the following allergens: A) Ole e 1, B) Ole e 2, C) Ole e 5 and D) Ole e 9.

4. Discussion and conclusions

The allergen content of the olive pollen is clearly influenced by the genetic origin of the cultivar analyzed (Hamman Khalifa et al. 2008). Diverse authors have also indicated that climatic factors may have different effects over olive flowering and pollen development (Galan et al. 2001; Orlandi et al. 2010), as well as over olive pollen allergenicity (Fernández-Caldas et al. 2007).

The results presented here demonstrate that changes occur in the expression of four relevant allergens in seven cultivars, and throughout consecutive years. However, results are considered heterogeneous between the different cultivars. The climatic parameters taken into account were temperature, precipitation, number of days of rain or relative humidity during the months prior to the flowering period, which normally corresponds to the months of May and June.

As regard to the temperature, correlations were not observed for a particular month or for the accumulated yearly temperature in all cultivars in a simultaneous way. However, the point correlations detected always corresponded to the winter and summer months (January-June) prior to the flowering period. This can be due to the intrinsic characteristics and requirements of each cultivar, or to the low number of cultivars and years studied, which may limit the statistical power of the analysis.

This results are in good agreement with those described for the birch major pollen allergen Bet v 1 (Buters et al. 2008), where an increase of this allergen was observed in higher temperatures, determined by growth of sampling trees in different climatic regions, over two consecutive years. Another study suggests a higher allergenic response to the Bet v 1 allergen present in birch pollen extracts grown in high average daily temperatures, in comparison to trees cultivated at lower temperatures (Ahlholm et al. 1998). This assay was carried out by using sera from patients sensitive to this pollen by using immunoblotting experiments. Our results indicate that high temperatures also seem to exert an increase in the expression of allergens in certain olive cultivars.

We may extrapolate that an increase in the average temperatures would bring a parallel increase in pollen allergenic content and allergenicity as a consequence. This could be therefore one of the consequences of the so-called global warming produced by the greenhouse effect (Ahlholm et al. 1998; Cecchi et al. 2010). Moreover, we may speculate that the fact that urban areas are often exposed to temperatures 2 to 8 °C higher that rural areas (Oke 1987) may result in increased olive pollen allergenicity and allergy prevalence in and around the cities, where the olive tree is also present, as it is widely used as an ornamental plant.

Fernández-Caldas et al. (2007) performed a similar study using six olive cultivars, over a period of five consecutive years. This study analyzed the content in the olive pollen major allergen (Ole e 1) only, which did not show statistically significant correlations to the precipitation average, nor to the average temperatures over the winter months prior to flowering. These authors described, however, a positive correlation between overall allergenicity and the average precipitation occurred during the winter months, for all the cultivars analyzed.

Several relevant differences are noticeable between the present study and that of Fernández-Caldas et al. (2007). First, this work combines the information available on four allergens, Ole e 1, Ole e 2, Ole e 5 and Ole e 9, instead of the olive pollen major allergen only. Therefore, the conclusions obtained are more similar to those described by Fernández-Caldas et al. referring to whole olive pollen allergenicity than those referring to Ole e 1 only. On the other hand, the present study uses accumulated data instead of averages for parameters like precipitation and number of monthly/seasonal/yearly days of rain. Moreover, although in some cases, monthly averages of temperature and relative humidity were considered, specific correlations were calculated upon the accumulated data for seasonal/yearly periods.

From an allergenic point of view, the present results suggest that those years with high levels of precipitation and high temperatures during the winter and the spring periods, contribute an enhanced allergenic content of the pollen grains at the end of the spring. We also may postulate that those areas of olive culture which are supplemented by artificial watering may yield a higher allergenicity for olive pollen-sensitized patients. The same would apply to urban areas, where ornamental olive trees are usually watered.

From an agronomic point of view, the described increase in the expression of the allergen Ole e 1 which takes place under increased temperature and precipitation might result in important differences in the reproductive behavior of the plant. Thus, preliminary observations (Morales et al. unpublished), indicated that the enhanced levels of Ole e 1 correlated to increased rates of pollen germination and lower degree of olive self-incompatibility. This hypothesis is also in good agreement with experimental observations made by several authors as regard to the effects of climatic factor on self-pollination and productivity in the olive (Androulakis and Loupassaki 1990, Lavee et al. 2002).

Author details

Sonia Morales
Proteomic Research Service, Hospital Universitario San Cecilio, Granada, Spain
Estación Experimental del Zaidín (CSIC), Granada, Spain

Antonio Jesús Castro, María Isabel Rodríguez-García and Juan de Dios Alché
Estación Experimental del Zaidín (CSIC), Granada, Spain

Acknowledgement

This work was supported by the Spanish Ministry of Science and Innovation (MICINN) (ERDF-cofinanced projects AGL2008-00517, BFU2011-22779 and PIE-200840I186) and the Junta de Andalucía (ERDF-cofinanced projects P2010-CVI5767 and P2010-AGR6274). The authors acknowledge the availability of plant material and the collaboration of the staff of the IFAPA center "Venta del Llano" (Mengíbar, Spain) depending from the Andalusian Regional Government.

5. References

Ahlholm, J.U., Helander, M.L., & Savolainen, J. (1998). Genetic and environmental factors affecting the allergenicity of birch (Betula pubescens ssp. czerepanovii [Orl.] Hamet-ahti) pollen. Clinical and Experimental Allergy, Vol. 28, No. 11, pp. 1384-1388, ISSN 1365-2222

Androulakis, I.I., & Loupassaki, M.H. (1990). Studies on the self-fertility of some cultivars in the area of Crete. *Acta Horticulturae*, Vol. 286, pp. 159-162, ISSN 0567-7572

Buters, J.T., Kasche, A., Weichenmeiera, I., Schober, W., Klaus, S., Traidl-Hoffmann, C., Menzel, A., Huss-Marp, J., Krämer, U., & Behrendt, H. (2008). Year-to-year variation in release of Bet v 1 allergen from birch pollen: evidence for geographical differences between West and South Germany. *International Archives of Allergy & Immunology*, Vol. 145, No. 2, pp. 122-130, ISSN 1018-2438

Cecchi, L., D'Amato, G., Ayres, J.G., Galan, C., Forastiere, F., Forsberg, B., Gerritsen, J., Nunes, C., Behrendt, H., Akdis, C., Dahl, R., & Annesi-Maesano, I. (2010). Projections of the effects of climate change on allergic asthma: the contribution of aerobiology. *Allergy*, Vol. 65, No. 9, pp. 1073-1081, ISSN 0105-4538

Fernández-Caldas, E., Carnés, J., Iraola, V., & Casanovas, M. (2007). Comparison of the allergenicity and Ole e 1 content of 6 varieties of Olea euroapea pollen collected during 5 consecutive years. *Annals of Allergy, Asthma & Immunology*, Vol. 98, No. 5, pp. 464-470, ISSN 1081-1206

Galan, C., Cariñanos, P., Garcia-Mazo, H., Alcazar, P., & Dominguez-Vilches, E. (2001). Model for forecasting *Olea europaea* L. airborne pollen in South-West Andalusia, Spain. *International Journal of Biometeorology*, Vol. 45, No. 2, pp. 59-63, ISSN 0020-7128

Hamman Khalifa, A.M., Castro, A.J., Rodríguez García, M.I., & Alché, J.D (2008). Olive cultivar origin is a major cause of polymorphism for Ole e 1 pollen allergen. *BMC Plant Biology*, Vol. 8, No. 10, ISSN 1471-2229

Lavee, S., Taryan, J., Levin, J., & Haskal, A. (2002). Importancia de la polinización cruzada en distintas variedades de olivo cultivadas en olivares intensivos de regadío. *Olivae: revista oficial del Consejo Oleícola Internacional*, Vol. 91, pp. 25-36, ISSN 0255-996X

Oke, T.R. (1987). Boundary Layer Climates. 2nd. Edition. London: Routledge. 435 pp.

Orlandi, F., Sgromo, C., Bonofiglio, T., Ruga, L., Romano, B., & Fornaciari, M. (2010). Spring Influences on Olive Flowering and Threshold Temperatures Related to Reproductive Structure Formation. *HortScience*, Vol. 45, No. 7, pp. 1052-1057, ISSN: 0018-5345

Morales, S., Castro, A.J., Jiménez-López, J.C., Florido, F., Rodríguez-García, M.I., & Alché J.D. (2012). A novel multiplex method for the simultaneous detection and relative quantification of pollen allergens. *Electrophoresis*, Vol. 33, pp. 1-8, DOI 10.1002/elps.201100667, ISSN: 1522-2683

Rabilloud, T., Vuillard, L., Gilly, C., & Lawrence, J.J. (1994). Silver-staining of proteins in polyacrylamide gels: a general overview. *Cellular and Molecular Biology (Noisy-le-Grand, France)*, Vol. 40, No. 1, pp. 57-75, ISSN 1165-158X

Chapter 5

Differential Immune-Reactivity and Subcellular Distribution Reveal the Multifunctional Character of Profilin in Pollen as Major Effect of Sequences Polymorphism

Jose C. Jimenez-Lopez, Sonia Morales, Dieter Volkmann, Juan D. Alché and María I. Rodriguez-Garcia

Additional information is available at the end of the chapter

http://dx.doi.org/10.5772/46170

1. Introduction

Profilin was first identified in plants as a birch allergen (Valenta et al. 1991). Plants have several genes encoding highly divergent profilin isoforms (Kovar et al. 2000; Kandasamy et al. 2002), differentially expressed, and with biochemical and functional diversity (Huang et al. 1996), particularly physiological roles in actin-based processes. Profilins are divided in two classes: one is ubiquitously present, and constitutively expressed in all plant tissues (vegetative), whereas the second class is restricted to the reproductive tissues (Kandasamy et al. 2002). At biochemical level, plant profilins are placed into two distinct classes: Class I profilins bind to phosphatidylinositol 4,5-bisphosphate [$PtdIns_{(4,5)}P_2$] much stronger than class II profilins, whereas class II have stronger affinity for actin and PLP (Gibbon et al 1998; Kovar et al 2000).

The complexity of profilin expression and the number of isoforms in higher plants is correlated with the observation that the actin family is also more complex in plants than in other kingdoms (McDowell et al. 1996). Structurally, Overall look to plant profilins indicates that they are similar to these from yeast and vertebrate, though the identity of primary amino acid sequence is only about 30% (Fedorov et al. 1997; Thorn et al. 1997), which implicate profilins in key conserved functions throughout different kingdoms. However, the *in vitro* biochemical data suggested that different profilin isoform functions distinctly (Kovar et al. 2000), which supports an isovariant dynamics model where particular isoforms have differential functions/activities. Supporting this idea, it has been proposed that plant profilin family multi-functionality might be inferred by natural variation through profilin isovariants generated among germplasm, as a result of polymorphism. The high variability might result in both differential profilin properties and differences in the regulation of the interaction with natural partners, suggesting that isovariant dynamics may expand the responses of the actin cytoskeleton or buffer it to against stress (Jimenez-Lopez 2008, Jimenez-Lopez et al. 2012).

Profilin is a major regulator of actin dynamics and is crucial for cellular growth, morphogenesis and cytokinesis (Jockusch et al. 2007). In addition to binding to actin, profilins bind to other partners like stretch of poly-proline (PLP) and proline-rich proteins, and phospholipids. The proline-binding ability could be a major function, being different among profilin isoforms, affecting actin-based structures (Kovar et al. 2001). The importance of the binding of profilin to PLP is supported by the finding of the differential preference for profilin isoforms of formin (essential actin-binding and nucleator protein) (Neidt et al. 2009), together with the evidence that *Arabidopsis* formins have preference for different profilin isoforms (Deeks et al. 2005).

Another binding ligand of profilin is phospholipids. The binding of profilin to phospholipids links to its potential role in vesicle trafficking (Janssen and Schleicher 2001). Profilins have been revealed as key mediators of the membrane–cytoskeleton communication, acting at critical points of signaling pathways initiated by events in the plasma membrane and transmitted by transduction cascades to promote cytoskeletal rearrangements (Baluska et al. 2002). This functionality arises from their capacity of interaction with phosphatidylinositides (PIP2), as well as with poly-L-proline-rich proteins (Kovar et al. 2001).

Several locations have been attributed to profilin. They have been localized in different plant cells and tissues, including the microspores, pollen grains and pollen tubes (Grote et al. 1993, 1995; Hess et al. 1995; Fischer et al. 1996; Vidali & Hepler 1997; Kandasamy 2002). Plant profilin was reported to be localized in the cytoplasm of pollen tube uniformly (Hess et al. 1995; Vidali & Hepler 1997). However, no clear picture has yet been established about the precise location of profilin in the pollen tubes. In consideration of the existence of calcium gradient in pollen tube and the regulation of profilin's sequestering activity by calcium (Kovar et al. 2000), the existence of a gradient of total sequestering activity of profilin in the pollen tube is expected.

Upon pollen hydration and pollen germination, profilin was detected close to the site of pollen tube emergence, forming a ring-like structure around the apertural region. Profilin was also detected in the pollen exine of the germinating pollen grains and in the germination medium. Profilin was also localized in the cytoplasm of the pollen tube, particularly at both the proximal and apical ends (Morales et al. 2008).

Depending on the fixation and extraction protocol used, nuclear localization has been also observed (Buss et al. 1992). Profilin has also been found in generative and vegetative nuclei of *Ledebouria socialis* pollen (Hess and Valenta 1997), the nuclei of *Phaseolus vulgaris* cells (Vidali et al. 1995) and *Arabidopsis thaliana* and maize root hairs (Braun et al. 1999, Baluska et al. 2001). Microinjection of a fluorescently labeled birch profilin in *Micrasterias denticulata* also shows an accumulation of profilin in the nucleus (Holzinger et al. 1997).

Other different profilin localizations have been described, like the chloroplast outer membrane, which interacts with CHUP1 protein during chloroplast movement in response to light (Schmidt von Braun and Schleiff 2008), and in amyloplasts (Fischer et al. 1996), in addition to a preferential localization in association with the plasma membrane. Moreover, a differential expression of different profilin isoforms has been reported in microspores and maize pollen (von Witsch et al. 1998). Profilin isoforms PRF1 and PRF2 were localized differentially in *Arabidopsis* epidermal cell (Wang et al. 2009), which emphasizes the existence of differentially regulated and localized profilin isoforms, as well as the necessity to determine the localization of each profilin isoform individually and carefully.

In the present study, we have used two experimental approaches: immune-reactivity in blotting experiments, and immunogold experiments for profilin cellular localization at TEM, with the aim of analyzing the differential immune-reactivity of profilins as result of their high sequence polymorphism, which also drives profilins the subcellular locations.

2. Material and methods

2.1. Plant material

Olive (*Olea europaea* L.) pollen was individually collected during May and June from olive trees of 24 cultivars, grown in the olive germplasm collection of the Estación Experimental del Zaidín, CSIC, Granada, Spain. Pollen samples were collected in large paper bags by vigorously shaking the inflorescences sequentially sieved through 150 and 50 μm mesh filters to eliminate debris and maintained at -80°C.

Mature seeds from Acebuche (wild olive) and Picual cultivars were obtained from the same collection of well-characterized olive trees growing in the "Estación Experimental del Zaidín" (Granada, Spain), 210 days after anthesis (DAA).

2.2. In vitro pollen germination

Olive mature pollen from the Picual cultivar was *in vitro* germinated. Pre-hydration was performed by incubation in a humid chamber at 30°C for 30 min. The grains (0.02 g/plate) were then transferred to Petri dishes containing 10mL of the germination medium [10% (w/v) sucrose, 0.03% (w/v) $Ca(NO_3)_2$, 0.01% (w/v) KNO_3, 0.02% (w/v) $MgSO_4$ and 0.03% (w/v) boric acid], as described by M'rani-Alaoui (2000). The Petri dishes were maintained at 25°C in the dark, and the pollen samples were taken at 5 min, 1, 4, 7, and 18h after the onset of the culture, pollen tube growth was monitoring by light microscopy. Finally, the pollen was pelleted by centrifugation (1000 × g for 20 s).

2.3. Protein extraction

Mature pollen or germinated samples were re-suspended in an extraction buffer (PBS), pH 7.4 [140 mM NaCl, 2.7 mM KCl, 8.15 mM Na_2HPO_4 and 1.8 mM KH_2PO_4] added with 10 μg/μL protease inhibitor cocktail (Sigma, Madrid, Spain) to a proportion of 5 mL solution per 0.5 gram of fresh tissue and then incubated at 4◦C for 4 h with vigorous shaking. After centrifugation at 13000 × g for 30 min at 4◦C, the supernatants were removed, dispensed into aliquots and stored at –20°C. The process was repeated two times and proteins from both protein extractions were precipitated together overnight at -20°C with a trichloroacetic acid solution.

0.5 g of seeds material (cotyledons and endosperms) was directly homogenized to a very fine powder in a liquid nitrogen-precooled mortar with a pestle. 0.1g of this powder was resuspended in 5ml of 1M Tris-HCl buffer, pH 7 plus 0.7% sodium dodecyl sulfate (SDS) and 1% 2-mercaptoethanol (denaturing, reducing conditions). After centrifugation at 10000*g* for 15 min (4°C), the supernatants were filtered through 0.2mm filter and stored at –20◦C.

The protein concentration was measured following the Bradford (1976) method, using the Bio-Rad reagent and bovine serum albumin (BSA) (Bio-Rad, Barcelona, Spain) as standard. In total, 30 μg of protein per lane was loaded into a 12% sodium dodecyl sulfate (SDS)-polyacrylamide gel (PAGE), as described by Laemmli (1970). The proteins were separated using a Mini-Protean system (Bio-Rad). After completion of SDS-PAGE, the gels were fixed and Coomassie blue stained [25% methanol, 10%acetic acid and 0.1% Coomassie blue R250]. Digitized images were obtained using the Power Look III scanner and the MagicScan software (UMAX Systems GmbH, Germany).

2.4. Protein transference and immunoblotting

After completion of proteins separation by SDS-PAGE, they were transferred onto polyvinylidenedifluoride (PVDF) membranes at 25 V for 30 min in a semi-dry transfer cell (Bio-Rad) with transfer buffer containing 25 mM Tris-HCl pH 8.3, 192 mM, and 20% glycine. For immunodetection, blots were incubated for 4 h at 25◦C with a blocking solution containing 0.1% Tween 20 and 10% dried skimmed milk in Tris-buffered saline (TBS). The membranes were then probed with:

1. Whole olive and maize profilins polyclonal antibodies anti-ZmPRA (dilution 1:500) and anti-Ole e 2 (Morales et al. 2008) in a dilution 1:20000.
2. Polyclonal antibodies specific to particular isoforms of maize profilin like ZmPRO5 (Kovar et al. 2000), ZmPRO4 (Gibbon *et al.* 1998) and ZmPRO3 (Karakesisoglou *et al.* 1996), in a dilution 1:500.

An alkaline phosphatase-Conjugated anti-rabbit IgG (Promega Co) diluted 1:10000 served as the secondary antibody, and the detection reaction was developed using NBT-BCIP colorimetric system.

2.5. Quantitations

The intensity of each band was calculated from scanned images of gels by using the quantitation tools of the Quantity One v4.6.2 software (Bio-Rad Laboratories, USA).

2.6. Microscopy analysis

2.6.1. Immunolocalization of profilins in pollen by Transmission Electron Microscopy

The germinated pollen grains were fixed for 2 h at 4°C in 0.1% (v/v) glutaraldehyde (GA) and 4% (w/v) parformaldehyde (PF) in buffer 1. The samples were dehydrated in an ethanol series and embedded in Unicryl resin (BBInternational, Cardiff, UK) following a progressive lowering of temperature (PLT) schedule, as described by Alché *et al.* (1999). Ultra-thin sections (80 nm) were cut with an ultramicrotome (Reichert- Jung, Vienna, Austria) and transferred on to formvar-coated 300-mesh nickel grids. Blocking of non-specific binding sites was carried out by incubation of sections for 2 h in a solution containing 5% (w/v) BSA in washing buffer. The blocking was followed by washing in buffer 1 for 10 min and incubation at RT for 2.5 h with the antibodies described above, and their proper dilutions in the blocking solution. After washing several times with buffer 1, the grids were treated for 2 h with a goat anti-rabbit IgG secondary antibody coupled to 15-nm gold particles (BBInternational) diluted 1/100 in the blocking solution. Finally, they were washed in buffer 1 (5 × 5 min), rinsed in double-distilled water (3 × 5 min) and then stained for 15 min with a solution of 5% (w/v) uranyl acetate in the dark. The observations were carried out with a JEM-1011 (JEOL, Tokyo, Japan) TEM. The treatment of control sections was the same, although incubation with the primary antibody was omitted.

2.7. Statistical analysis

Statistical analysis was performed by using the SPSS v.18 statistical software package. A general comparison among multiple sample groups was performed throughout one-way analysis of variance (One-way ANOVA) on the basis of the Fisher-Snedecor distribution test (α=0.05, significance value) (Mehta and Patel 1983). Normality and variances homogeneity of the data collection were checked by the Shapiro-Wilk test (α= 0.05, significance value) (Shapiro and Wilk 1965) and the Levene test (α= 0.05 significance value) (Levene 1960), respectively. Post hoc range probes and pair of species comparisons were carried out with the parametric test of Games-Howell (α=0.05, significance value) (Games and Howell 1976).

3. Results

3.1. Expression and differential reactivity characterization of profilin from olive cultivars

SDS-PAGE analysis of protein extracts of mature pollen from 24 olive cultivars showed distinctive protein profiles with different intensity.

30μg of total protein was loaded in each line. The main protein bands of know pollen allergens correspond to the mayor olive pollen allergen Ole e 1, with a molecular weigh between 18-20 kDa. Defined protein bands corresponding to profilin around 13-15kDa are not clearly distinguishable (Figure 1).

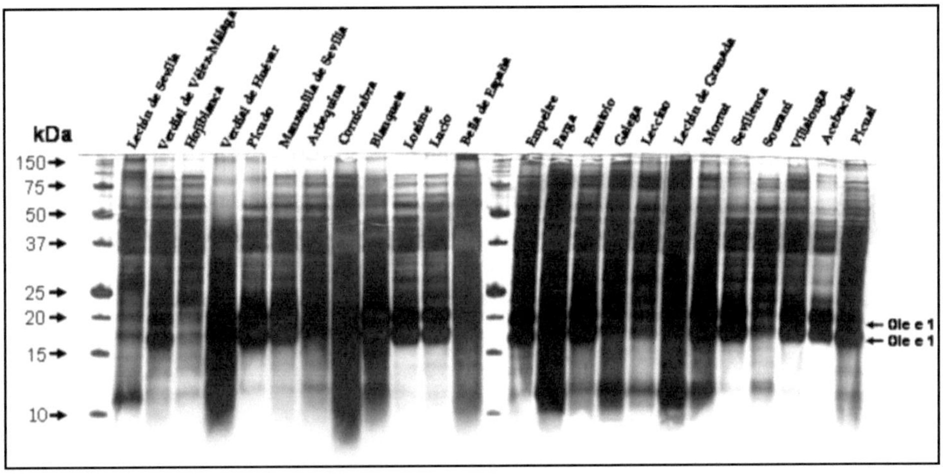

Figure 1. Protein profile of crude protein extract from 24 olive cultivars.

Cross-reactivity analysis between protein extracts from 24 olive cultivars with different antisera made against profilins from olive and maize pollen showed large differences both qualitative (intensity of bands) and quantitative (number of reactive bands) concerning profilins of MW around 13, 13.7 y 14.2kDa (Figure 2).

Statistical analysis of densitometric quantitations was performed. The variance analysis for the different antisera against different protein extracts from 24 olive cultivars (Figure 2 A to E) showed significant differences (F-ratio=14.06, $p<0.05$). The reactivity values were inside a normal distribution (Shapiro-Wilk=0.85, $p>0.05$), while the Levene test indicated non homogeneity of variances (Levene=10.16, $p<0.05$).

Multiple comparisons of the five antisera by Games-Howell test determined the existence of statistically significant differences ($p<0.05$) between pairs of serum analyzed (anti-PRA to anti-ZmPRO4, anti-PRA to anti-ZmPRO3, anti-ZmPRO4 to anti-ZmPRO5, and anti-ZmPRO3 to anti-ZmPRO5, with Games-Howell test results of 73705.4, 70384.6, 124308.1 and 53923.4, respectively.

The analysis of the reactivity of the different cultivars against each individual antiserum showed statistical significant differences between Leccino and Picual, Lechín de Sevilla and Picudo, Lucio and Frantoio, Blanqueta and Farga, as well as between Picudo and Cornicabra corresponding to the immunoblots individually probed with anti-PRA, anti-ZmPRO3, anti-ZmPRO5, anti-ZmPRO4 y anti-Ole e 2, respectively (Figure 2A-E). Oppositely, it is possible to observe clear differences between antisera in their reactivity to defined cultivars, such as Hojiblanca, Arbequina, Cornicabra, Bella de España and Empeltre for the immunoblotting corresponding to anti-ZmPRO3; Lechin de Sevilla, Verdial de Huevar, Loaime, Lucio and Leccino for anti-ZmPRO4; and Sourani and Villalonga for anti-Ole e 2 (Figure 2A-E).

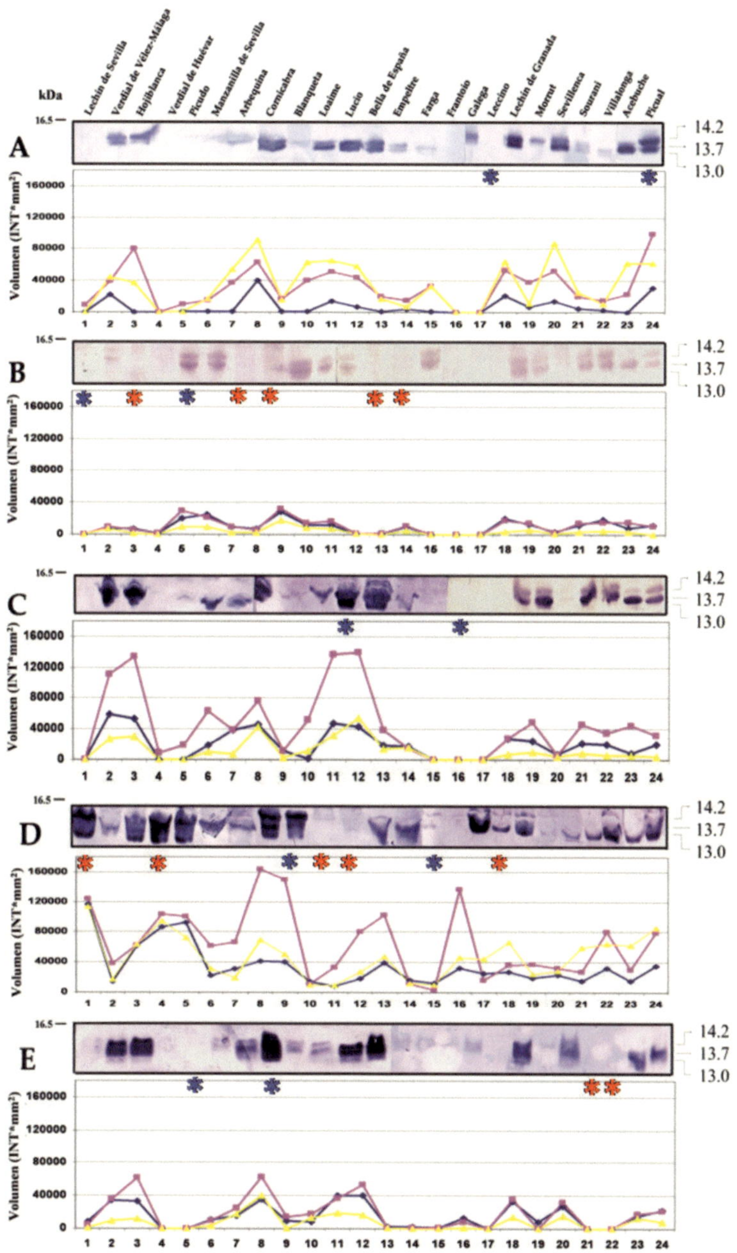

Figure 2. Immuno-reactivity analysis of profilin from 24 olive pollen cultivars. Reactivity of protein crude extracts from 24 olive cultivars was assayed against different maize profilin antisera, A) anti-PRA, B) anti-ZmPRO3, C) anti-ZmPRO5, D) anti-ZmPRO4, E) as well as against olive profilin antiserum anti-Ole e 2. Up to 3 reactive bands about 13, 13.7 and 14.2 kDa, corresponding to different isoforms of profilins were observed. The intensity of the reactive bands was quantitated by a densitometric analysis: yellow plot corresponding to 13kDa bands, pink (13.7 kDa) and blue (14.2 kDa). Red asterisks highlighted the differential reactivity (very high or very low) of defined cultivars to particular antisera, whereas blue asterisks highlighted the differential reactivity among cultivar to defined antisera.

3.2. Profilin expression and characterization of the differential reactivity of birch, hazel, timothy-grass and maize profilins

SDS-PAGE analysis of protein extracts of mature pollen from *Betula pendula, Corylus avellana, Phleum pratense* and *Zea mays* displayed distinctive protein profiles in the figure 3. Defined protein bands corresponding to profilin are clearly distinguishable in the interval of 14-17kDa, which is the expected size for profilin isoforms.

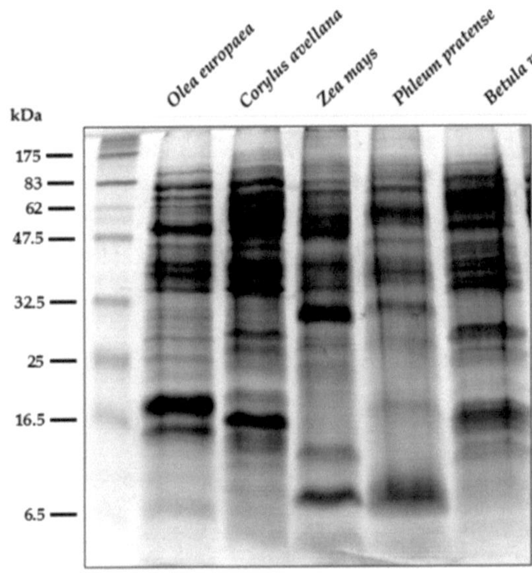

Figure 3. Protein profile of crude protein extract from pollen of 5 individual plant species. 30μg of total protein was loaded in each line.

Profilin immunodetection was performed by using the same antisera described above for olive. In this case, different antisera are able to distinguish up to two reactive bands, with molecular weights of 13.7 and 14.2 kDa (Figure 4).

Clear differences can be appreciated when compared protein extracts reactivity of different species to individual antisera, as well as the reactivity of an individual protein extract to the different antisera assayed.

Cross-immune reactivity analysis between protein extracts from the five species with different antisera made against profilins from olive and maize pollen showed large differences both qualitative (intensity of bands) and quantitative (number of reactive bands) concerning profilins of MW around 13.7 and 14.2 kDa (Figure 4).

Statistical analysis of densitometric quantitations was performed. The variance analysis for the different antisera against different protein extracts showed significant differences among the 5 species (F-ratio= 8.13, $p<0.05$).

The reactivity values were inside of a normal distribution (test de Shapiro-Wilk: 0.95, $p>0.05$), while the Levene test indicated non-homogeneity of variances (Levene: 2.86, $p<0.05$).

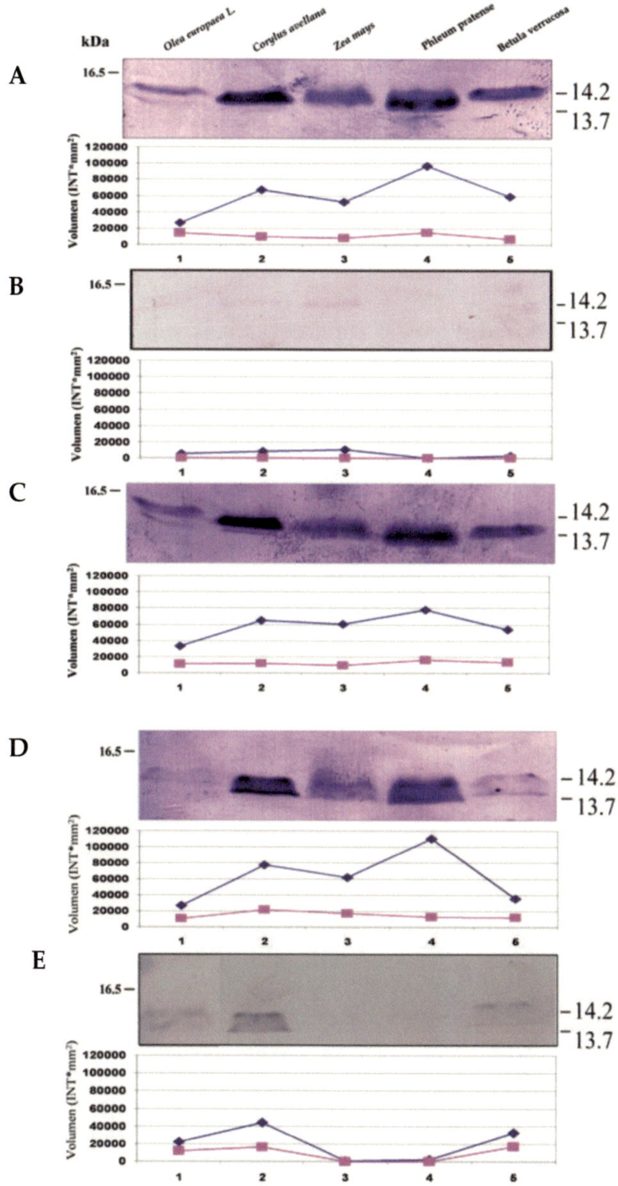

Figure 4. Immuno-reactivity analysis of crude protein extract from pollen of 5 plant species. Reactivity of proteins from 5 plant species were assayed against different maize profilin antisera, A) anti-PRA, B) anti-ZmPRO3, C) anti-ZmPRO5, D) anti-ZmPRO4, E) as well as against olive profilin antiserum anti-Ole e 2. It was appreciable up to 2 reactive bands about 13.7 and 14.2 kDa, corresponding to different isoforms of profilins for the species analyzed. The intensity of the reactive bands was quantitated by a densitometric analysis: pink color plot corresponded to 13.7kDa bands, and blue to 14.2 kDa. Red asterisks highlighted the differential reactivity (very high or very low) of defined species to different antisera, whereas blue asterisks highlighted the differential reactivity among cultivar to defined antiserum.

Multiple comparison among the antisera showed statistically significant differences ($p<0.05$) between anti-ZmPRO3 and anti-PRA, anti-ZmPRO4, and anti-ZmPRO5, respectively, with Games-Howell test results of 65010.5, 64564.3 y 71150.2, respectively.

On the other hand, analysis of reactivity among species against individual antiserum showed statistical significant differences between *Olea europaea* L. and *Phleum pratense*, *Olea europaea* L. and *Corylus avellana*, *Zea mays* and *Phleum pratense*, and *Corylus avellana* and *Zea mays* for the antisera anti-PRA, anti-ZmPRO5, anti-ZmPRO4 and anti-Ole e 2, respectively.

Reversely, it is possible to observe clear differences between antisera for defined species, such as *Corylus avellana* and *Phleum pratense* for anti-ZmPRO3, and *Phleum pratense* for anti-Ole e 2.

3.3. Analysis of olive pollen profilin during *in vitro* germination

The study of the olive pollen germination was aimed to analyze the differential expression of profilin isoforms during the germination process. Figure 5 showed the protein profiles of olive pollen extracts (cv. Picual) obtained after hydration, and at different times of germination (5 min, 1h, 4h, 7h and 18h). No bands were distinguishable in the blue Coomassie blue stained gel around the molecular weight corresponding to profilins.

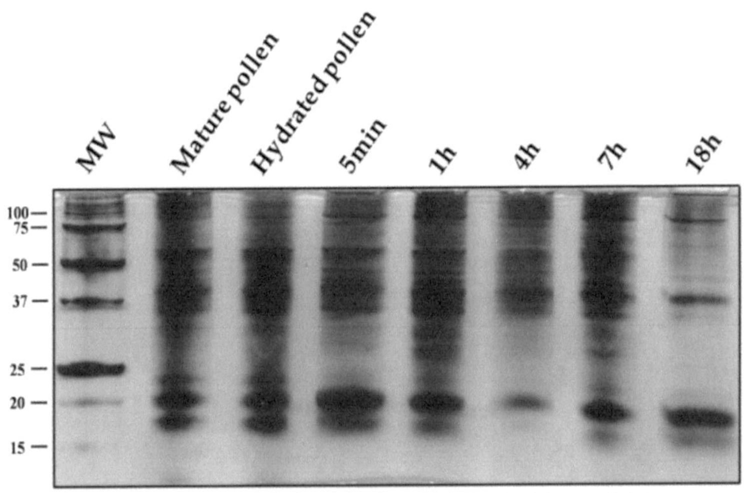

Figure 5. Protein profile of crude protein extract of mature olive pollen (cv. Picual) before and at different times of *in vitro* germination. 30μg of total protein was loaded in each line.

On the contrary, clear bands were obtained with immunoblotting experiments with the different antisera. 5 different bands can be distinguished corresponding to 5 different profilin isoforms (Figure 6), with calculated MW of 13.0, 13.7, 14.2, 14.9 and 15.7 kDa, respectively.

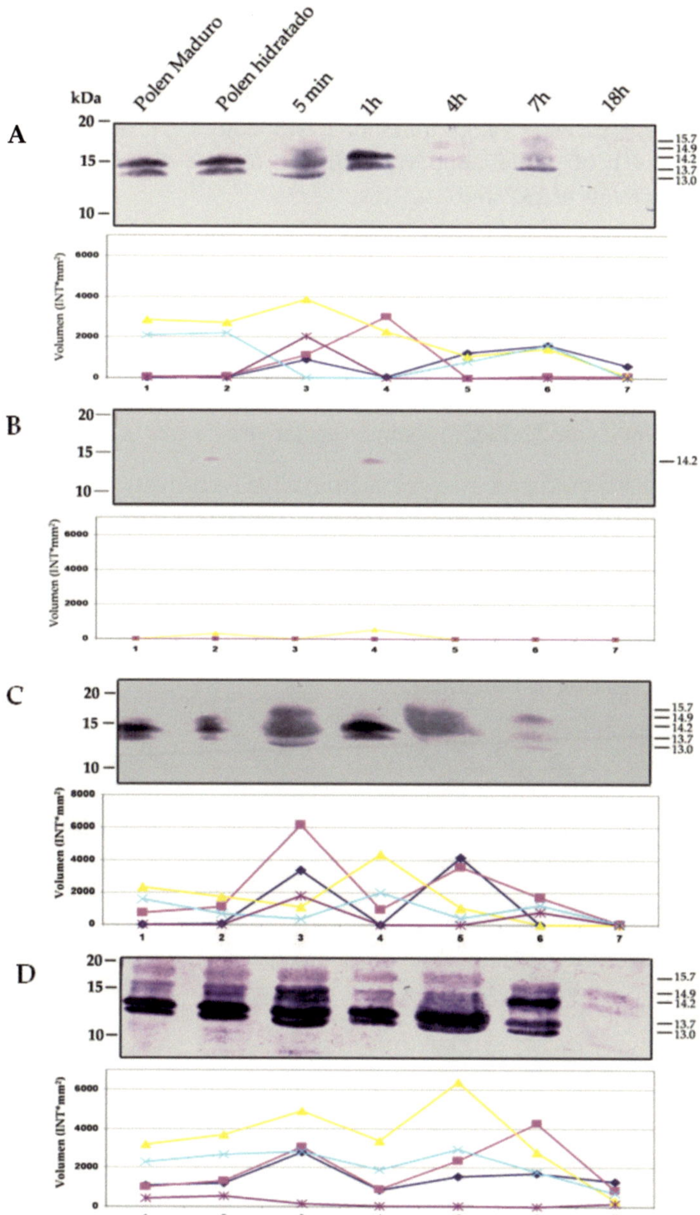

Figure 6. Immune-reactivity analysis of crude protein extract of mature olive pollen (cv. Picual) before and after *in vitro* germination. Reactivity of proteins extracts from mature pollen, as well as different stages of *in vitro* germination were assayed against different maize profilin antisera, a) anti-PRA, b) anti-ZmPRO3, c) anti-ZmPRO5, d) anti-ZmPRO4, e) as well as against olive profilin antiserum anti-Ole e 2. It was appreciable up to 5 reactive bands about 13.0, 13.7, 14.2, 14.9 y 15.7 kDa, corresponding to different isoforms of profilins. The intensity of the reactive bands was quantitated by a densitometric analysis: blue color plot corresponded to 13.0kDa bands, pink, yellow, turquoise, and brown color to 13.7, 14.2, 14.9 and 15.7 kDa, respectively.

The expression pattern of profilin is similar during *in vitro* germination, although conspicuous differences of the antisera reactivity can be pointed out for the protein extracts. Level of protein isoforms expression in mature pollen and hydration stage were quite similar. On the other hand, there was a notable decrease of protein expression level, equally for all the isoforms at the end of germination (7-18 hours). Proteins expression level between 5 min and 4 h of germination was variable for the different profilin isoforms, particularly for the variants of 13.7 and 14.2 KDa.

3.4. Analysis of cross-immunoreactivity between vegetative and reproductive profilins

In order to determine the putative cross-reaction between reproductive profilins (see sections 3.1 to 3.3) and profilins from vegetative tissues, we have tested two of the antibodies used above (anti-ZmPRO4, and anti-ZmPRO5) against vegetative isoforms of maize profilins.

For this purpose, we have used protein extracts from olive seeds (cotyledon and endosperm) (cv Picual and Acebuche). The analysis of olive seed proteins Figure 7A showed a protein profile completely different to these of protein extracts from pollen. In this case, the mayor protein bands corresponded to different polypeptides of seed storage proteins, with MW ranging from 20 to 47kDa (Alché et al. 2006).

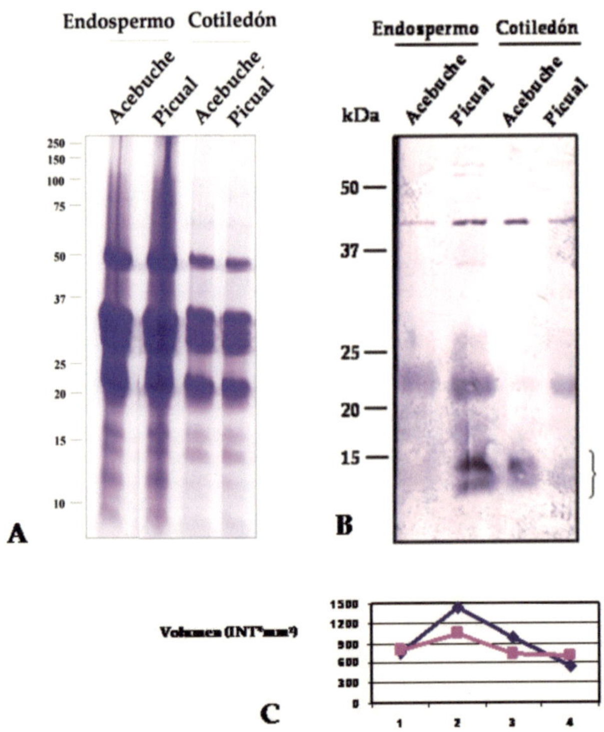

Figure 7. Immune-reactivity analysis of crude protein extract of vegetative profilins from olive seed tissues, cotyledon and endosperm.

The immunoblotting analysis of seed proteins with anti-Ole e 2 showed at least two reactive bands located at 13.7 and 14.2 kDa (Figure 7B). In addition, there were quantitative differences in the expression level of profilin concerning both tissues (cotyledon and endosperm) and cultivar. Thus, profilin in endosperm of cultivar Picual showed a higher level of immune-reactivity in comparison with profilins of cotyledon from the same cultivar.

Protein extracts from olive seed cultivars Acebuche and Picual were used in immunoblot experiments with antiserum anti-Ole e 2. A) SDS-PAGE of crude protein extract from olive seeds tissues (endosperm and cotyledon) of Acebuche and Picual cultivars. B) Inmunoblot of seeds protein samples from (A). Reactive bands were observed at 13.7 and 14.2 kDa, corresponding to vegetative profilins. C) Plot corresponding to the quantitation of reactive bands: blue lines were depicted for 14.2 kDa bands, whereas pink color was used for 13.7 kDa reactive bands.

Specie	Sequence GeneBank Accession N°	Chloroplast	Mitochondria	Secretory Pathway	Others (Cytoplasm, Microsomes)
Olea europaea L.	-	**13.2±1.6**	**8.2±0.8**	**9.8±0.5**	**68.8±0.7**
	DQ640909	5.9±0.0	4.4±0.0	39.9±0.0	49.8±0.0
	DQ640910	7.6±0.0	7.0±0.0	20.0±0.0	65.4±0.0
	DQ640906	5.8±0.0	5.3±0.0	32.2±0.0	56.7±0.0
	DQ640903	9.7±0.0	7.4±0.0	14.2±0.0	68.7±0.0
	DQ640908	7.9±0.0	7.8±0.0	17.0±0.0	67.3±0.0
	DQ317580	6.7±0.0	4.8±0.0	28.4±0.0	60.1±0.0
	DQ640904	8.2±0.0	6.8±0.0	15.2±0.0	69.8±0.0
	DQ663553	6.7±0.0	4.8±0.0	28.4±0.0	60.1±0.0
	DQ663554	6.7±0.0	4.8±0.0	28.5±0.0	60.0±0.0
	DQ663555	6.9±0.0	4.4±0.0	28.2±0.0	60.5±0.0
	DQ663556	6.7±0.0	4.8±0.0	28.5±0.0	60.0±0.0
	DQ663558	8.7±0.0	6.8±0.0	20.0±0.0	64.5±0.0
	DQ640905	7.1±0.0	8.4±0.0	16.5±0.0	68.0±0.0
	DQ60907	8.2±0.0	6.8±0.0	15.3±0.0	69.7±0.0
Betula pendula	-	**14.4±1.1**	**8.6±0.5**	**11.7±0.3**	**65.3±1.0**
Corylus avellana	-	**14.4±0.1**	**8.1±0.1**	**13.2±0.5**	**64.6±0.4**
	DQ663545	8.4±0.0	6.8±0.0	22.3±0.0	62.5±0.0
	DQ663547	6.5±0.0	4.2±0.0	27.7±0.0	61.6±0.0
Phleum pratense	-	**6.6±0.2**	**5.0±0.3**	**27.9±0.7**	**61.5±1.4**
Zea mays	-	**7.8±0.1**	**7.2±0.1**	**19.7±0.4**	**65.4±0.4**
	X73280	2.5±0.0	9.9±0.0	27.1±0.0	60.5±0.0

Table 1. Score calculated for the probability of finding a specific profilin in a particular cellular location. Bold numbers indicate that the score calculated for these sequences markedly differed from the average value.

3.5. Cellular localization of profilin

3.5.1. Predicting the cellular localization of profilin

Predictions of the cellular location for profilins were carried out based in their primary sequence, and the putative presence of signal peptides responsible for targeting these proteins to specific cellular locations.

Probability of profilins location was calculated by using the tools TargetP (www.cbs.dtu.dk) and v2.0 PSORT (psort.hgc.jp). Table 1 shows the average values of probability for profilins location in different cellular compartments.

Overall, profilins exhibited high probability for cytoplasm localization. However, some sequences had a significant score for being localized in mitochondria and chloroplasts, while others were targeted to the secretory pathway. These data were confirmed by the program SignalP 3.0 Server (www.cbs.dtu.dk) (results not shown).

In addition, it was calculated the average probability of nuclear localization of profilins in the table 2, where different sequences from species exhibited a higher or lower probability of localization in comparison with an average score. Based in the average score, profilins from *Olea europaea* L. are most likely localized in nucleus compared with the other species.

Plant profilins analyzed have a targeting motif for nuclear localization which sequence is (RGKKGXGG(I/V)T(I/V)KKT) (Yoneda 1997).

Specie	Sequence GenBank Accession N°	Probability of Nuclear Location (%)
Olea europaea L.	-	**34.8±3.3**
	DQ138337	19.0±0.1
	DQ138325	18.0±0.1
	DQ117904	19.0±0.1
Betula pendula	-	**25.5±0.7**
Corylus avellana	-	**29.1±0.8**
	DQ663545	17.0±0.1
Phleum pratense	-	**27.8±1.5**
	X77583	33.0±0.1
	Y09546	32.0±0.1
	Y09457	31.0±0.1
	Y09458	32.0±0.1
Zea mays	-	**26.9±2.0**
	X73279	32.0±0.1
	X73280	35.0±0.1

Table 2. Score of probability for nuclear distribution of profilins. Bold numbers indicate the average probability.

The polymorphism of the profilin sequences concerning this motif is depicted in the table 3. Overall, micro-heterogeneities in this motif were identified for several sequences of olive, hazel and timothy-grass. These changes can represent differences in the affinity for localization of particular profilin isoforms in defined cellular locations.

Specie	Sequence GeneBank Accession N°	Nuclear Targeting Motif	Specie	Sequence GeneBank Accession N°	Nuclear Targeting Motif
	DQ640909	RGKKGAGGITIKKT	*Corylus avellana*	DQ663545	RGKKGAGGITVKKT
	DQ640910	RGKKGAGGITVKKT		DQ663547	RGKKGAGGITVKKT
	DQ138336	RGKKGAGGITIKKT		X77583	RGKKGAGGITIKKT
	DQ640906	RGKKGAGGITIKKT		Y09546	RGKKGAGGITIKKT
	DQ640908	RGKKGAGGITVKKT		Y09457	RGKKGAGGITIKKT
	DQ317574	RGKKGSGGITSKKT		Y09458	RGKKGAGGITIKKT
	DQ663553	RGKKGAGGITIKKT		DQ663535	RGKKGAGGITIKKT
Olea europaea L.	DQ663554	RGKKGAGGITIKKT	*Phleum pratense*	DQ663536	RGKKGAGGITIKKT
	DQ663555	RGKKGAGGITIKKT		DQ663537	RGKKGAGGITIKKT
	DQ663556	RGKKGAGGITIKKT		DQ663538	RGKKGAGGITIKKT
	DQ663557	RGKKGAGGITIKKT		DQ663539	RGKKGAGGITIKKT
	DQ640905	RGKKGAGGITVKKT		DQ663540	RGKKGAGGITIKKT
	DQ138358	RGKKGTGGITIKKT		DQ663541	RGKKGAGGITIKKT
	DQ138352	RGKKGSGGITIKET		DQ663542	RGKKGAGGITIKKT
	DQ138354	RGKKGSGGITIKET			

Table 3. Changes in the motif targeting to a nuclear localization of profilin sequences.
Sequence of nuclear motif is characterized by the sequence RGKKGXGG(I/V)T(I/V)KKT, where X is the amino acid serine (**S**) in the majority of the analyzed sequences. The variable amino acids were highlighted in bold and red color.

3.5.2. Experimental approach for profilin cellular localization

The experimental approach for profilin localization was performed to determine whether there is really a differential distribution of profilin isoforms. Immuno-localization assays were performed by transmission electron microscopy (TEM) in ultrathin sections of germinated pollen grains of olive (cv. Picual) using different antisera: anti-Ole e 2 and anti-PRA (Figures 8 and 9), anti-ZmPRO3 (Figure 10), anti-ZmPRO4 (Figure 11), anti-ZmPRO5 (Figure 12).

All immune-localizations showed that profilins (gold particles) were preferentially located in the cytoplasm (Figures 8A and 9-12A), in addition to both nuclei of vegetative/generative cell (Figures 8A and 9A). Moreover, abundant gold grains were located in the pollen apertures (Figures 8C, 10C and 11C), in along the pollen wall, pollen tube and the pollen tip (Figures 8A and 9-12B), as well as in the material associated with the pollen grain exine (pollen coat) (Figures 8B, 11B and 12C). No significant number of labeling were found in the negative controls, for which were omitted the primary antiserum (Figure 9C). The overall number of gold grains in the sections was variable, and depending on the antiserum used.

Profilin distribution					
Antiserum	Cytoplasm	Pollen Coat	Aperture	Negative Control	Pollen Germination Media
Anti-PRA	6.06±3.94	7.83±4.67	8.22±2.22	2.00±0.42	27.13±8.89
Anti-ZmPRO3	34.70±9.66	8.83±4.54	4.86±2.04	5.00±0.87	48.56±23.76
Anti-ZmPRO4	5.91±3.02	4.34±1.32	10.83±3.06	2.00±0.38	32.75±9.63
Anti-ZmPRO5	13.00±3.35	5.14±1.95	2.20±0.45	3.00±0.44	18.70±17.36

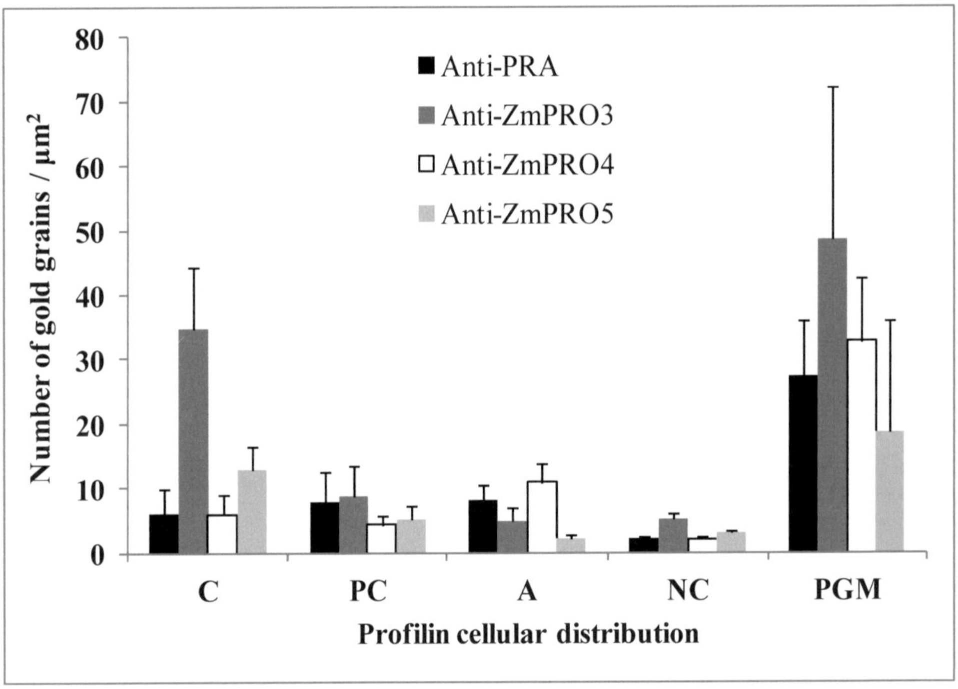

Table 4. Gold grains count for each antiserum used in this study. Measures corresponded to gold grains/μm². Profilin counting values corresponding to the different subcellular localization were plotted. **C**= Cytoplasm; **PC**= Pollen Coat; **A**= Aperture; **NC**= Negative Control; **PGM**= Pollen Germination Media.

In order to determine differences in the gold grain distribution for the different antisera used as markers for profilin isoforms, we proceeded to count the gold particles present on each of the above mentioned compartments. The results of this quantitation are showed in the table 4. The most abundant immunolabeling was observed in sections incubated with individual antiserum following the next order: anti-ZmPRO3 > ZmPRO4 > ZmPRO5. Antisera anti-ZmPRO5 and ZmPRO3 showed a preferential cytoplasmic immunolocalization, whereas anti-PRA and anti-ZmPRO4 showed a preferential localization in the apertural regions of the pollen grain.

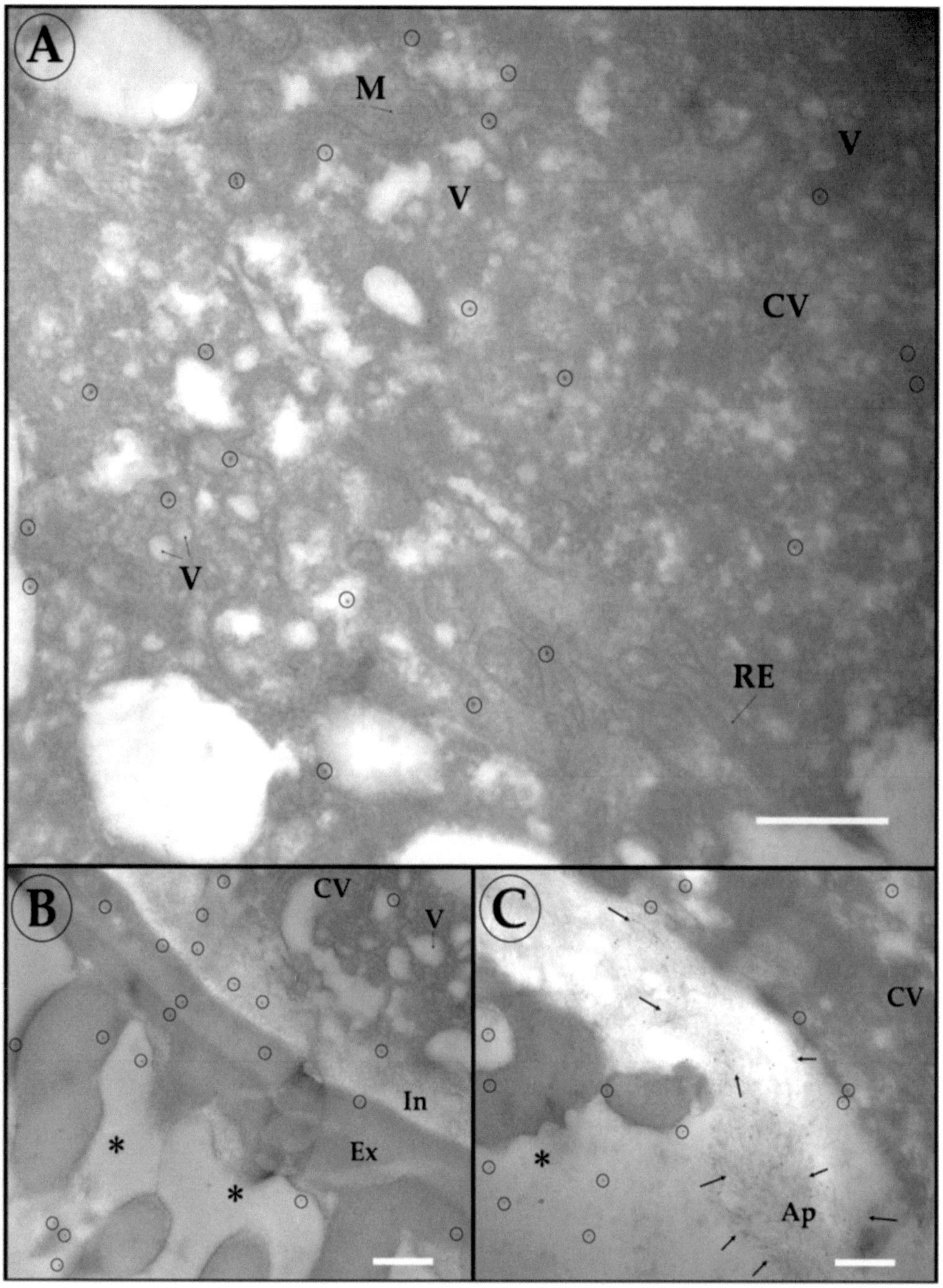

Figure 8. TEM immune-localization of olive pollen profilin in sections of mature pollen (cv Picual) during in vitro germination by using anti-Ole e 2 antiserum. A) General view of the vegetative cell cytoplasm, B) pollen grain walls C) and the apertural region. The location of the gold particles is highlighted with circles and arrows. Ap: apertures; CV: vegetative cell cytoplasm, Ex: exine, In: intine, M: mitochondria, N: nucleus, P: plastid, ER: endoplasmic reticulum; V: vesicle, asterisks: material adhered to the pollen walls (pollen coat). The bars represent 1 μm.

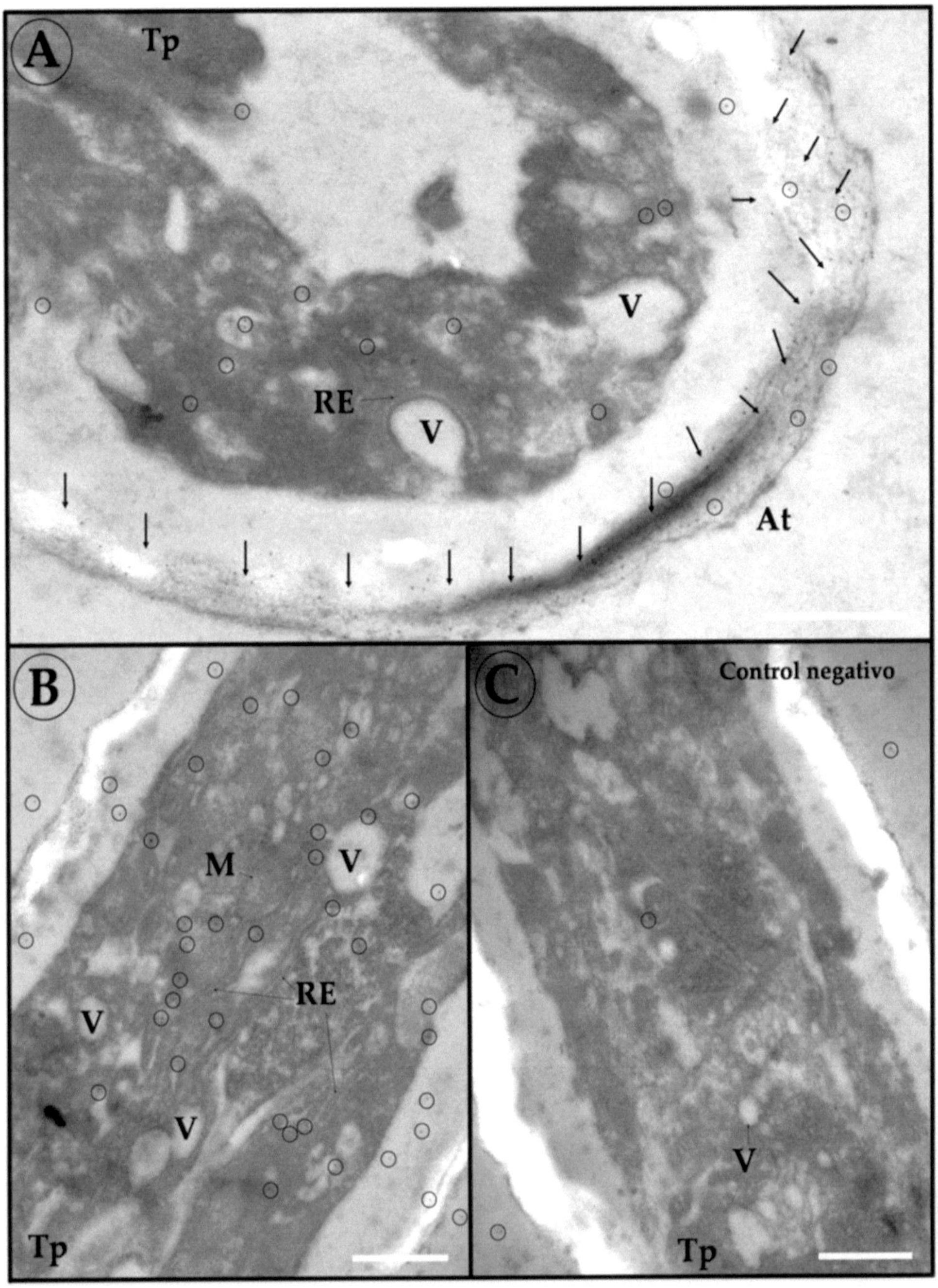

Figure 9. TEM immune-localization of olive pollen profilin in sections of mature pollen (cv Picual) during in vitro germination by using anti-PRA antiserum. A) General view of the pollen tip, B) longitudinal section of a pollen tube, and C) negative control. The location of the gold particles is highlighted with circles and arrows. Ap: apertures; CV: vegetative cell cytoplasm, Ex: exine, In: intine, M: mitochondria, N: nucleus, P: plastid, ER: endoplasmic reticulum; Tp: pollen tube; V: vesicle, asterisks: pollen coat. The bars represent 1 μm.

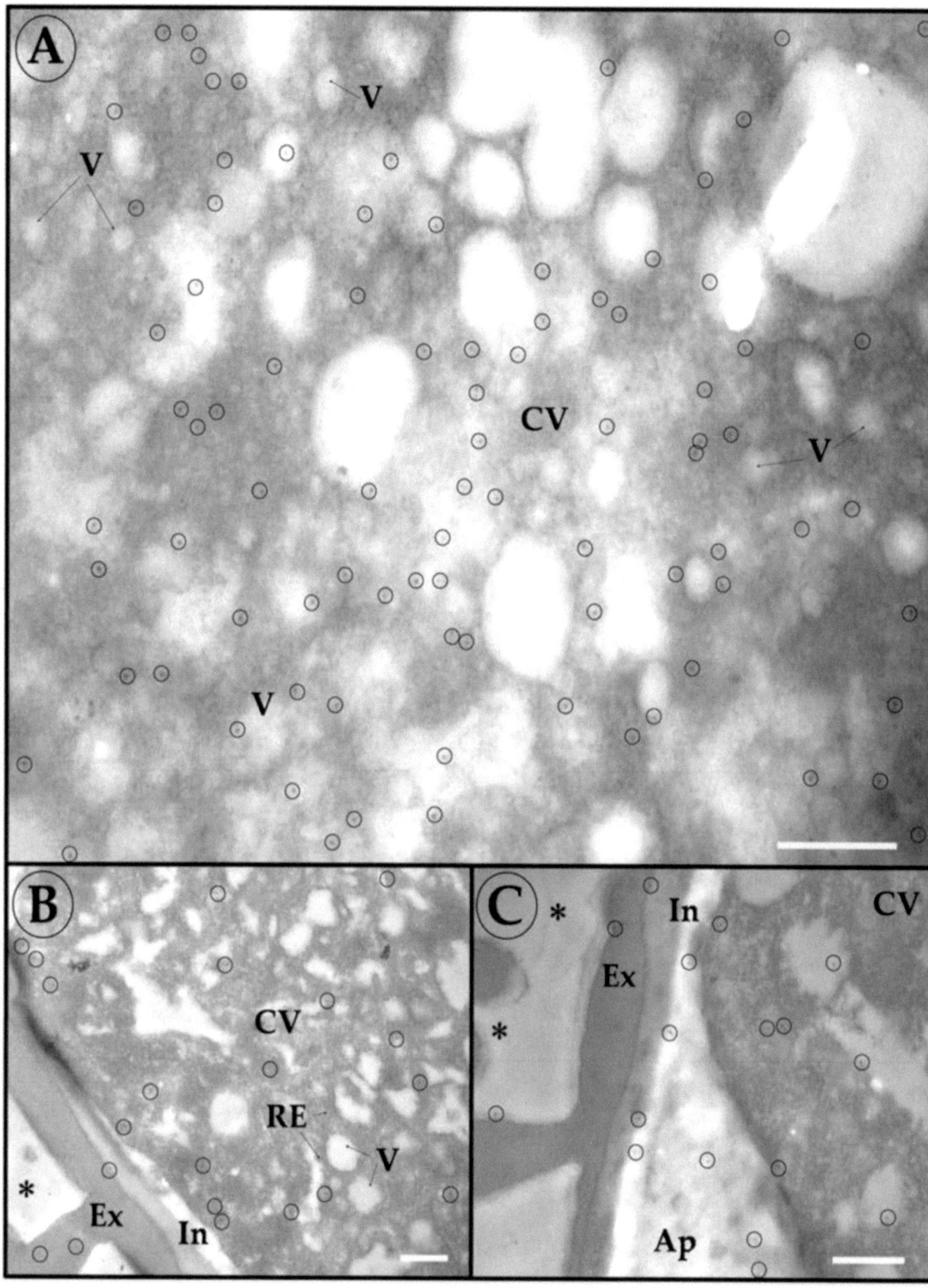

Figure 10. TEM immune-localization of olive pollen profilin in sections of mature pollen (cv Picual) during in vitro germination by using anti-ZmPRO3 antiserum. A) General view of the vegetative cell cytoplasm, B) pollen grain walls, and C) apertural region. The location of the gold particles is highlighted with circles and arrows. Ap: apertures; CV: vegetative cell cytoplasm, Ex: exine, In: intine, M: mitochondria, N: nucleus, P: plastid, ER: endoplasmic reticulum; V: vesicle, asterisks: pollen coat. The bars represent 1 μm.

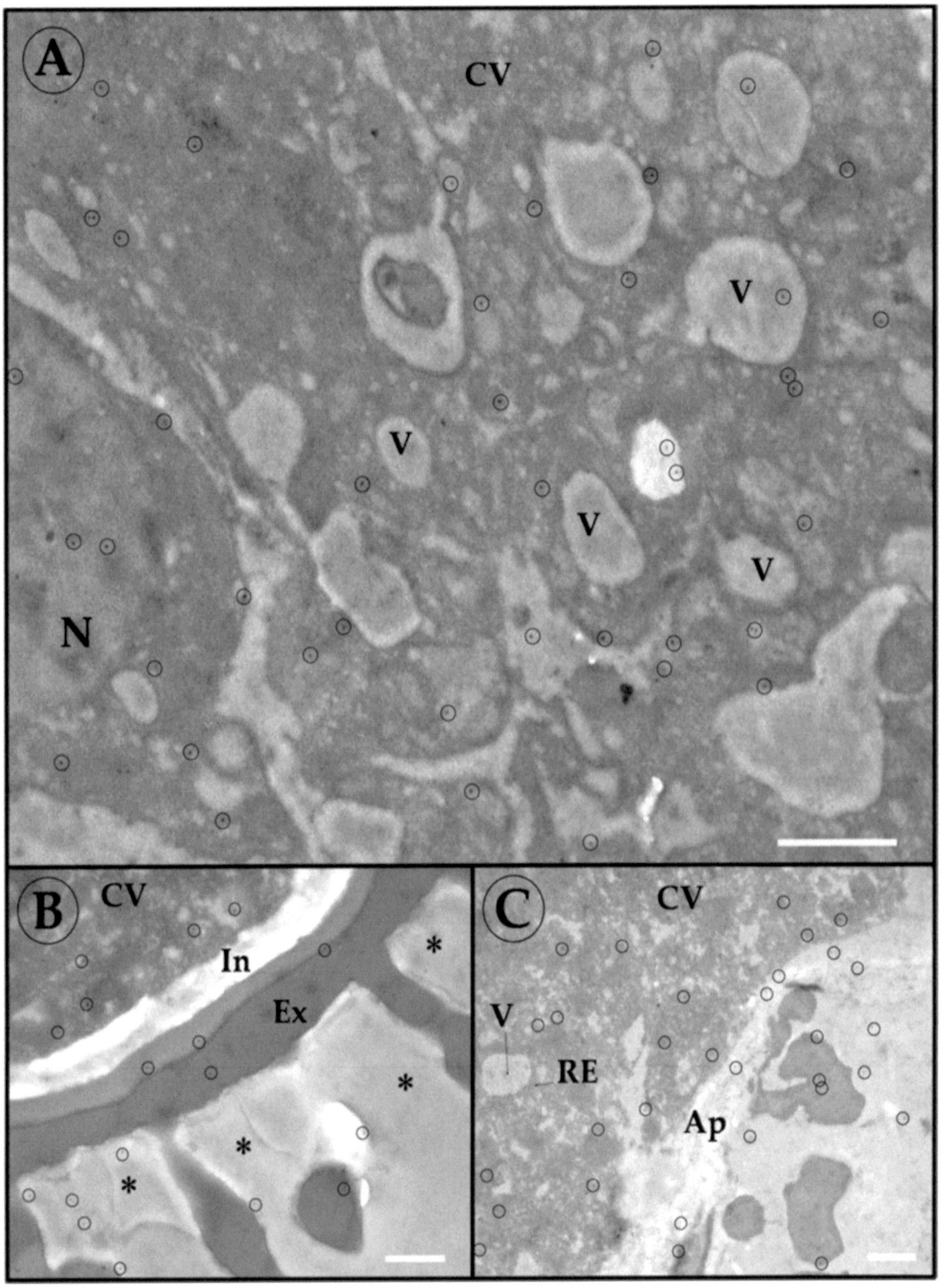

Figure 11. TEM immune-localization of olive pollen profilin in sections of mature pollen (cv Picual) during in vitro germination by using anti-ZmPRO4 antiserum. A) General view of the vegetative cell cytoplasm, B) pollen grain walls, and C) apertural region. The location of the gold particles is highlighted with circles and arrows. Ap: apertures; CV: vegetative cell cytoplasm, Ex: exine, In: intine, M: mitochondria, N: nucleus, P: plastid, ER: endoplasmic reticulum; V: vesicle, asterisks: pollen coat. The bars represent 1 μm.

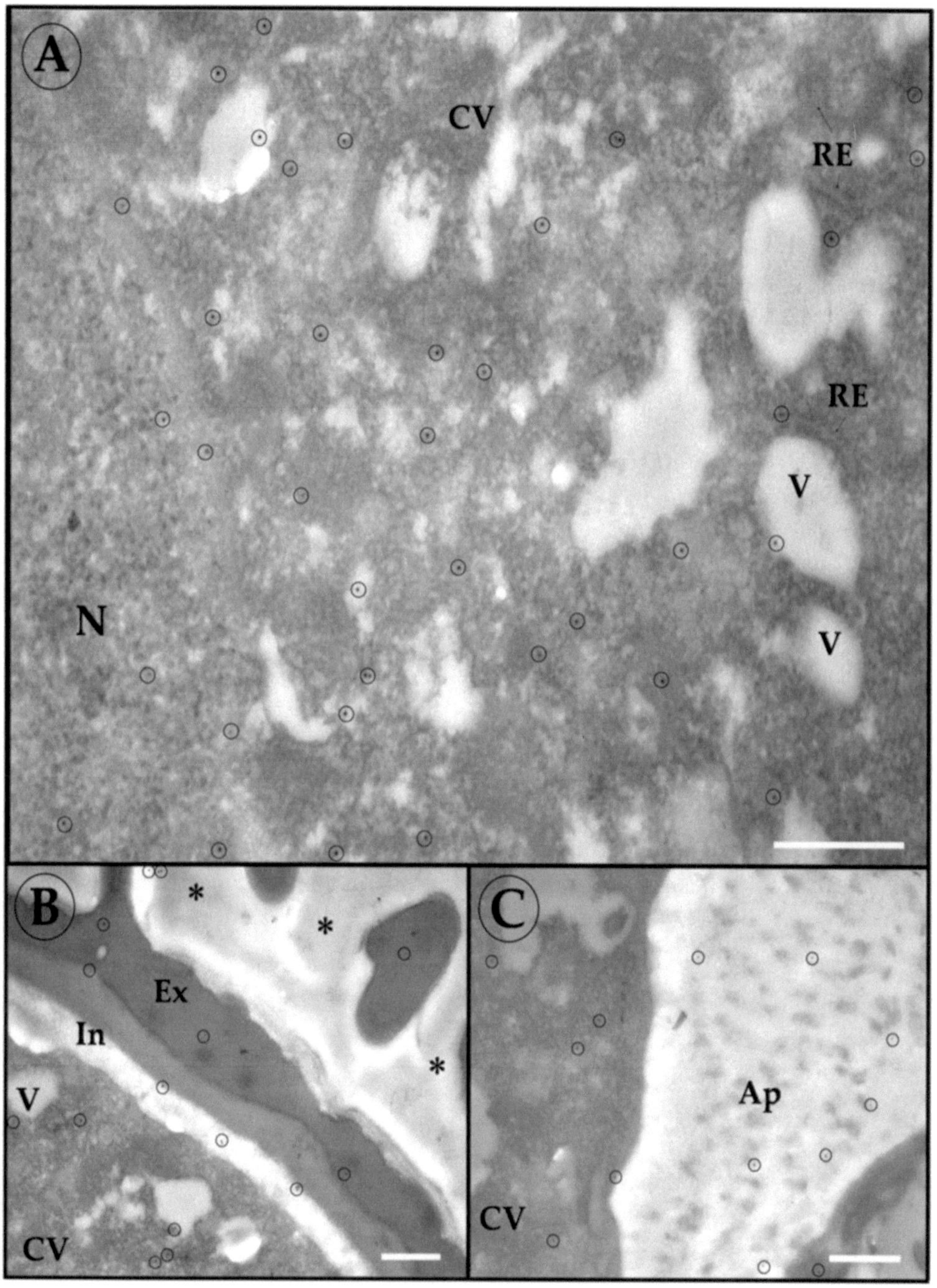

Figure 12. TEM immune-localization of olive pollen profilin in sections of mature pollen (cv Picual) during in vitro germination by using anti-ZmPRO5 antiserum. A) General view of the vegetative cell cytoplasm, B) pollen grain walls, and C) apertural region. The location of the gold particles is highlighted with circles and arrows. Ap: apertures; CV: vegetative cell cytoplasm, Ex: exine, In: intine, M: mitochondria, N: nucleus, P: plastid, ER: endoplasmic reticulum; V: vesicle, asterisks: pollen coat. The bars represent 1 μm.

4. Discussion

4.1. Molecular characteristics of profilin explain the pan-allergen character and their specific cross-immune reactivity

Profilins as pan-allergens are present in a wide variety of plant sources, and responsible for numerous cross-reactions. On the other hand, profilins are also able to elicit allergic responses highly specific by recognition of specific epitopes (immuno-dominant regions of recognition and interaction with B cells and T of the human immune system). IgE antibody production by B lymphocytes IgE-mediated response plays a major role in cross-reactivity between allergens and the symptoms of allergy (Aalberse et al. 1992). However, in addition to humoral responses, has been shown that the cross-reactivity also attends through humoral responses mediated by T cells, i.e. reactivity to allergens of plant foods (Mal d 1, Api g 1 and Dau c 1) with the pollen allergen Bet v 1. In the first case, it is likely that both fresh and cooked food (in which conformational epitopes are lost), induce T cell activation and symptoms mediated by them, and do so in the absence of binding to IgE (Bohle et al. 2003). The allergenic responses (mechanisms) should be considered of special relevance, since knowledge gained on antigens recognized by T- and B-cells will allow a better understanding of specific immune responses with applications in allergy therapy (López-Torrejón et al. 2007).

The "double allergenic activity" of profilin can be explained by the combination of a high structural conservation, together with the presence of a high sequence polymorphism.

The experimental results clearly demonstrate that different forms of profilins have described differential immunological characteristics as they respond differently to the antibodies used. This suggests that the recognition of profilins by the human immune system would also very likely to be differential. Several reasons can justify the broad cross-reactivity of the different profilins:

1. The presence of a number of specific and common surface features in the structure of the majority of allergens can make differences in immune-reactivity among allergens. Typically, a high hydrophobicity of amino acids integrating epitopes, in addition to good accessibility to the region of the protein seems to be key parameters for high reactivity,
2. The epitopes more relevant in determining the reactivity of the profilins are conformational epitopes, not linear. Thus special consideration should be given to the potential electrostatic and solvent exposure of these molecules in order to find out what the specific IgE epitopes responsible for cross-reactions.
3. Secondary structural elements of the proteins such as regions rich in α-helices, β sheets or turns are factors promoting that reactivity. These characteristics have been observed not only in profilin, but also in other families such as LTP and allergenic storage proteins of seeds (Seong & Matzinger 2004). Moreover, the similarities between the structure of human and grasses profilins in addition to other different plant species

might be a cause of the possible role of human profilin in the extension of allergic symptoms caused by profilins of other species in atopic patients (Valenta et al. 1991).

4. Another relevant factor described as a possible cause of cross-reactions in multiple species, even if they are phylogenetically distant, is the presence of polymeric forms of allergens, i. e. plant and human profilin (Valenta et al. 1994). Vrtala et al. (1996) have shown that birch profilin induced an IgG response, subclass 2 (IgG2) in mice and primates, which is typical of polymeric antigens. Maize profilin isoform ZmPRO1 can be in multimeric forms that persist even after denaturing and reducing agents in similar manner that happens with the native human profilin (Babich et al. 1996). In addition, the formation of profilin multimers is not incompatible with the profilin function/activity carried out through interaction with its ligands (Jonckheere et al. 1999). Differential recognition of plant profilin multimers by the immune system is not based in a simple additive effect, because profilin multimers act synergistically to facilitate sterical access to binding sites which present unique epitopes (Psaradellis et al. 2000).
5. Cross-reactivity and pan-allergen character is not the only important feature that distinguishes profilins in their immune-reactivity. Several studies have documented very specific allergenic reactivity of the profilins. Some of these have shown that specific IgE epitopes can even distinguish variables plant profilins, even from the same family, and the reactivity among plant profilins is only partial (Vallverdu et al. 1998). These differences in reactivity can be attributed to the presence of a high polymorphism in these molecules (Radauer et al. 2006).

Polymorphism is a common feature in many allergenic proteins. It has been reported different degrees of polymorphism in diverse allergen sources, which include dust mites (Piboonpocanun et al. 2006), food (Hales et al. 2004, Gao et al. 2005) and pollen allergens of different tree species and herbaceous (Chang et al. 1999). However, although the polymorphism is beginning to be detailed in depth, relatively little is known about the causes which originate. In some cases, the allergen polymorphism has been attributed to the presence of multigene families (Bond et al. 1991). In other allergens, the presence of multiple forms of the allergen can be explained by the existence of posttranslational modifications (Batanero et al. 1996a). In apple (*Malus domestica*), have been characterized up to 18 genes of Mal d 1, and there is differences in allergenicity depending on the cultivar (Gao et al. 2005) which may be due to this extensive allelic diversity. In olive, it has been shown that polymorphism of the allergen Ole e 1 is clearly linked to genetic background (cultivar) (Hamman-Khalifa et al. 2008), similarly to what happens to Ole e 2, where there are differential molecular characteristics due to polymorphism, which would be sufficient to explain the differences in reactivity allergenic / immunogenic among profilins from different species, different olive varieties, and even among the same isoforms of profilins (Jimenez-Lopez 2008; Jimenez-Lopez et al. 2012).

The experimental data suggest that the profilin family of proteins likely contains numerous functionally-distinctive isoforms, also reflected in differential cellular localizations as a result of a differential expression of some forms of profilins in vitro germination of pollen grain, and the preferential localization of some forms of profilins in different cellular compartments. These data also revealed that the differential immune-reactivity of profilins is likely the result of the presence of both common and specific epitopes features, which would be generated by the described sequence polymorphism, and might explain differential sensitizations of allergenic patients to olive pollen cultivars as well as cross-reactions between pollens from different species, as well as pollen and food allergens.

In the present work, it has been identified up to five immune-reactive bands to antibodies in the different extracts analyzed, after separation of the polypeptides by electrophoresis. The number of bands identified in other studies (Alché et al. 2007) also ranges from 3 to 5, depending on the separation methods employed, and the observed molecular weight ranges are very similar.

It is noteworthy to see that there is differential reactivity of the profilins in different species (and varieties in the case of the olive tree) to the antibodies used in immunoblot experiments. These differences vary not only depending on the antibody used, but for a given antibody can be observed dramatic differences in the reactivity of a species (varieties), and even between different forms of profilins (different bands) within the same species or variety. These differences have proved to be statistically. These type of experiential evidences can highlight two important aspects that distinguish the immunological reactivity of profilins: i) profilins are responsible for cross-allergenicity between allergens (recognizable bands in almost all species and/or varieties) and ii) other antibodies are able to recognize subtle differences in the structure between different forms of these molecules (differences in the reactivity of protein bands between species and varieties with different antibodies). In this sense, the observed differences in the reactivity of the extracts of different varieties of olive, seems to support the varietal character as discriminatory parameter in pollen allergens, as clearly was demonstrated for other allergens such as Ole e 1 (Hamman-Khalifa et al. 2008), and Ole e 2 (Jimenez-Lopez 2008; Jimenez-Lopez et al. 2012) in the case of olive.

The cellular localization observed for profilins in this work corresponds essentially to that predicted by bioinformatics tools, which is otherwise very similar to that described by other authors. With a few exceptions (eg Fischer et al. 1996 that Phl p 4 located in amyloplasts of pollen from Phleum pratense), most authors reported the profilins localization in the cytoplasm and exine of pollen grain and in the cytoplasm of pollen tube. The olive pollen, profilins are found distributed in the cytoplasm of the pollen grain and pollen tube, without preferential localization or binding to organelles, structures or compartments. The large presence of labeling was also associated to the exine, the material adhered to the exine and the apertural region can be considered distinctive, suggesting evidences of a massive release of the allergen to the media when pollen is hydrated, which has been previously described for Ole e 2 and Ole and 1 (Alché et al. 2004; Morales et al. 2008).

Immunolocalization experiments using anti-ZmPRO4 and anti-ZmPRO5 confirm the predictions of nuclear localization for olive pollen profilins. Such accumulation may be the result of passive diffusion due to the small size of profilin that allows them to pass through the nuclear pore complex (Yoneda 1997). However, a possible active and selective process by a non-classical signal of nuclear localization, or perhaps other elements such as importin-like proteins might be implicated in that nuclear localization (Yoneda 1997). In animal cells, has been found exportin-like proteins that are specific for profilin (exportin 6) and recognizes only the actin-profilin complex, which export the complex outside the nucleus.

Furthermore, in the nucleus has been also located several natural ligands of profilin like PIP2 (Mazzotti et al. 1995), actin and other ABPs such as ADF-cofilin in maize (Jiang et al. 1997) and CAPG (Lu & Pollard 2001). Nuclear distribution suggests that profilin could play an important role in controlling the function of nuclear actin (Rando et al. 2000), in addition to be involved in processes such as chromatin condensation and translation signals from cytoplasm to nucleus (Valster et al. 2003).

4.2. Implications of polymorphism in the diagnosis and allergy therapy

Cross-reactivity between profilins has broad implications in the phenomena of allergy, being responsible for many cases of double sensitization to pollens and various foods (van Ree 2004). Furthermore, the high cross-reactivity might justify the current use of a single profilin (recombinant profilin of birch pollen, Bet v 2) for the diagnosis of allergy.

The existence of high polymorphism and differential reactivity to different profilin isoforms may have a number of consequences for the diagnosis and allergy therapy. Given the differential reactivity of patients to different forms of profilins, it is extremely important that the extracts used in clinical trials should take in consideration the existence of polymorphism in these molecules. As reviewed by Alché et al. (2007), the content of allergens in the protein extracts should be as similar as possible to the panel of proteins to which the atopic patient is usually exposed and reactive. Therefore, in the case of patients with allergy to profilins, it should be carefully analyzed their reactivity to the different isoforms, in order to adjust or "personalize" the treatment. In addition, a great advantage of this customization is the increased safety of immunotherapy treatments, avoiding undesirable sensitization induced “de novo” by immunotherapy, which have been documented by several authors.

New concepts in diagnosis and therapy often include the use of recombinant allergen molecules (Crameri and Rhyner 2006). Recombinant allergens undoubtedly provide tremendous advantages over the use of specific conventional allergen immunotherapy, based on the use of extracts from natural sources. However, a reduction in the number of allergen proteins in the extracts for immunotherapy (as is happening through the exclusive use of a single recombinant profilin form) may lead to the emergence of substantial differences between vaccines and the actual exposure of patients to their environments, unless a careful selection of the panel of recombinant allergens for immunotherapy is made. This strategy can be incorporated into virtually all new vaccines currently under development to improve the diagnosis and therapy, and to include the hybrid or modified molecules, allergen fragments, multimers, or the design of hypoallergenic proteins. For instance, a detailed reactivity analysis of isoforms present in particular cultivars, combined with protein sequence analysis, could aid the design of hypoallergenic proteins, which might complement the strategies currently in use (Marazuela et al. 2007). Besides a thorough investigation of the allergenic isoforms of the germplasm species could also help identifying natural hypoallergenic profilin isoforms in some cultivars of olive.

5. Conclusion

This study highlights and support a previous work developed by the same group (Jimenez-Lopez 2008; Jimenez-Lopez et al. 2012) about multi-functionality and regulatory importance evolved from sequence polymorphism of pollen profilins, as a potential mechanism to generate multiple profilin isovariants in a wide genetic (germplasm) background of particular plant species like olive.

This polymorphism in profilin isovariants is reflected in the differential immune-reactivity exhibited by different cultivars to antibodies generated against vegetative and reproductive profilins, in addition to differential subcellular location in pollen grains and germinated pollen tubes. Both characteristics lead to strongly propose that functional differences among profilin isoforms, as well as regulatory pathways throughout profilin-ligand binding properties, could have a direct influence in the subcellular location and actin cytosqueleton dynamics as direct consequence of polymorphism. Furthermore, this variability reflected in the epitopes generation in panallergen like Ole e 2, has extreme importance in the standardization of formulations for allergy diagnosis in clinical trials and tailored-immunotherapy development.

Author details

Jose C. Jimenez-Lopez, Sonia Morales,
Juan D. Alché and María I. Rodriguez-Garcia
Department of Biochemistry, Cell and Molecular Biology of Plants,
Estación Experimental del Zaidín, Spanish National Research Council (CSIC), Granada, Spain

Dieter Volkmann
Institute of Cellular and Molecular Botany (IZMB), Department of Plant Cell Biology,
University of Bonn, Germany

Acknowledgement

This study was supported by the following European Regional Development Fund co-financed grants: MCINN BFU 2004-00601/BFI, BFU 2008-00629, BFU2011-22779, CICE (Junta de Andalucía) P2010-CVI15767, P2010-AGR6274, P2011-CVI-7487, P2011-CVI-7487, and by the coordinated project Spain/Germany MEC HA2004-0094.

The funders had no role in the study, design or decision to publish.

6. References

Alché, J.D., Castro, A.J., Jimenez-Lopez, J.C., Morales, S., Zafra, A., Hamman-Khalifa, A.M., and Rodríguez-García M.I. (2007). Differential characteristics of olive pollen from different cultivars: biological and clinical implications. *Journal investigational allergology and clinnical immunology*, Vol. 17, Suppl. 1, pp. 17-23.

Alché, J.D., M'rani-Alaoui, M., Castro, A.J., & Rodríguez-García, M.I. (2004). Ole e 1, the major allergen from olive (*Olea europaea* L.) pollen increases its expression and is released to the culture medium during in vitro germination. *Plant and cell physiology*, Vol. 45, N°. 9, pp. 1149-1157.

Alché, J.D., Jimenez-Lopez, J.C., Wei, W., Castro-Lopez, A.J., and Rodríguez-García, M.I. (2006). Biochemical characterization and cellular localization of 11S type storage proteins in olive (*Olea europaea* L.) seeds. *Journal of Agricultural and Food Chemistry*, Vol. 54, pp. 5562-5570.

Aalberse, R.B. (1992). Clinically significant cross-reactivities among allergens. *International archives of allergy and immunology*, Vol. 99, pp. 261-264.

Babich, M., Foti, L.R.P., Sykaluk, L.L., and Clark, C.R. (1996). Profilin Forms Tetramers That Bind to G-Actin. *Biochemical and Biophysical Research Communications*, Vol. 218, N°. 1, pp. 125-131.

Baluška, F., Jasik, J., Edelmann, H.G., Salajová, T. and Volkmann, D. (2001). Latrunculin B-induced plant dwarfism: Plant cell elongation is F-actin-dependent. *Developmental biology*, Vol. 231, pp. 113-124.

Baluška, F., and Volkmann, D. (2002) Actin-driven polar growth of plant cells. *Trends in Cell Biology*, Vol. 12, N°. 1, pp. 14

Batanero, E., Villalba, M., Monsalve, R.I., and Rodríguez, R. (1996a). Cross-reactivity between the major allergen from olive pollen and unrelated glycoproteins: Evidence of an epitope in the glycan moiety of the allergen. *Journal of allergy and clinnical immunology*, Vol. 97, pp. 1264-1271.

Bohle, B., Radakovics, A., Jahn-Schmid, B., Hoffmann-Sommergruber, K., Fischer, G.F., and Ebner, C. (2003). Bet v 1, the major birch pollen allergen, initiates sensitization to Api g 1, the major allergen in celery: evidence at the T cell level. *European Journal of Immunology*, Vol. 33, N°. 12, pp. 3303 – 3310.

Bond, J.F., Garman, R.D., Keating, K.M., Briner, T.J., Rafnar, T., Klapper, D.G., and Rogers, B.L. (1991). Multiple Amb a I allergens demonstrate specific reactivity with IgE and T cells from ragweed-allergic patients. *Journal of Immunology*, Vol. 146, pp. 3380-3385.

Braun, M., Baluska, F., von Witsch, M., and Menzel, D. (1999). Redistribution of actin, profilin and phosphatidylinositol-4, 5-bisphosphate in growing and maturing root hairs. *Planta*, Vol. 209, pp. 435-443.

Buss, F., Temm-Grove, C., Henning, S., and Jockusch, B.M. (1992). Distribution of profilin in fibroblasts correlates with the presence of highly dynamic actin filaments. *Cell motility and the cytoskeleton*, Vol. 22, N°. 1, pp. 51-61.

Chang, Z.N., Peng, H.J., Lee, W.C., Chen, T.S., Chua, K.Y., Tsai, L.C., Chi, C.W., and Han, S.H. (1999). Sequence polymorphism of the group 1 allergen of Bermuda grass pollen. *Clinnical and experimental allergy*, Vol. 29, pp. 488-496.

Crameri, R., and Rhyner, C. (2006). Novel vaccines and adjuvants for allergen-specific immunotherapy. *Current opinion in immunology*, Vol. 18, N°. 6, pp. 761-768.

Deeks, M.J., Hussey, P.J., and Davies, B. (2002). Formins: intermediates in signaltransduction cascades that affect cytoskeletal reorganization. *Trends in Plant Science*, Vol. 7, pp. 1360–1385.

Fedorov, A.A., Ball, T., Valenta, R., and Almo, S.C. (1997). X-ray crystal structures of birch pollen profilin and Phl p 2. *International archives of allergy immunology*, Vol. 113, N. 1-3, pp. 109-113.

Fischer, S., Grote, M., Fahlbusch, B., Müller, W.D., Kraft, D., and Valenta, R. (1996). Characterization of Phl p 4, a major timothy grass (*Phleum pratense*) pollen allergen. *The Journal of allergy and clinical immunology*, Vol. 98, N°. 1, pp. 189-198.

Gao, Z.S., Weg, W.E., Schaart, J.G., Arkel, G., Breiteneder, H., Hoffmann-Sommergruber, K., & Gilissen, L.J. (2005). Genomic characterization and linkage mapping of the apple allergen genes Mal d 2 (thaumatin-like protein) and Mal d 4 (profilin). *Theoretical and applied genetics*, Vol. 111, N. 6, pp. 1087-1097.

Games, P.A., and Howell, J.F. (1976). Pairwise multiple comparison procedures with unequal n's and/or variances: A Monte Carlo study. *Journal of Educational Statistics*, Vol. 1, N°. 2, pp. 113–125.

Gibbon, B.C., Zonia, L.E., Kovar, D.R., Hussey, P.J., & Staiger, C.J. (1998). Pollen profilin function depends on interaction with proline-rich motifs. *Plant Cell*, Vol. 10, pp. 981-994; [Correction: *Plant Cell*, Vol. 11, pp. 1603]

Grote, M., Swoboda, I., Meagher, R.B., and Valenta, R. (1995). Localization of profilin and actin-like immune-reactivity in vitro-germinated tobacco pollen tubes by electron microscopy after special water-free fixation techniques. *Sexual Plant Reproduction*, Vol. 8, pp. 180–186.

Grote, M., Vrtala, S., and Valenta, R. (1993). Monitoring of two allergens, Bet v I and profilin, in dry and rehydrated birch pollen by immunogold electron microscopy and immunoblotting. *The journal of histochemistry and Cytochemistry*, Vol. 41, N. 5, pp. 745-750.

Hales, B.J., Bosco, A., Mills, K.L., Hazell, L.A., Loh, R., Holt, P.G., and Thomas, W.R. (2004). Isoforms of the major peanut allergen Ara h 2: IgE binding in children with peanut allergy. *International archives of allergy and immunology*, Vol. 135, pp. 101-107.

Hamman Khalifa, A., Castro, A.J., Jimenez-Lopez, J.C., Rodríguez García, M.I., and Alché, J.D. (2008). Olive cultivar origin is a major cause of polymorphism for Ole e 1 pollen allergen. *BMC Plant Biology*, Vol. 8, pp. 10

Hess, M.W., and Valenta, R. (1997). Profilin revealed in pollen nuclei: immuno-electron microscopy of high-pressure frozen *Ledebouria socialis* Roth (Hyacinthaceae). *Sexual Plant Reproduction*, Vol. 10, pp. 283–287.

Hess, M.W., Mittermann, I., Luschnig, C., and Valenta, R. (1995). Immunocytochemical localisation of actin and profilin in the generative cell of angiosperm pollen: TEM studies on high-pressure frozen and freeze-substituted *Ledebouria socialis* Roth (Hyacinthaceae). *Histochemistry and Cell Biology*, Vol. 104, N. 6, pp. 443-451.

Holzinger, A., Valenta, R., and Lütz-Meindl, U. (2000). Profilin is localized in the nucleus-associated microtubule and actin system and is evenly distributed in the cytoplasm of the green alga Micrasterias denticulata. *Protoplasma*, Vol. 212, pp. 197–205.

Huang, S.R., McDowell, J.M., and Weise, M.J., and Meagher, R.B. (1996). The Arabidopsis profilin gene family. Evidence for an ancient split between constitutive and pollen-specific profilin genes. *Plant Physiology*, Vol. 111, pp. 115–126.

Janssen, K.P., and Schleicher, M. (2001). *Dictyostelium discoideum*: a genetic model system for the study of professional phagocytes. Profilin, phosphoinositides and the lmp gene family in Dictyostelium. *Biochimica et biophysica acta*, Vol. 1525, N. 3, pp. 228-233.

Jiang, C.J., Weeds, A.G., and Hussey, P.J. (1997). The maize actin-depolymerizing factor, ZmADF3, redistributes to the growing tip of elongating root hairs and can be induced to translocate into the nucleus with actin. *Plant Journal*, Vol. 12, pp. 1035–1043.

Jimenez-Lopez, J.C. PhD Thesis 2008. Molecular characterization of profilin polymorphism in the pollen of olive and other allergogenic species. ISBN: 978-84-691-4573-9; DOI: 10481/1871

Jimenez-Lopez, J.C., Morales, S., Castro, A.J., Volkmann, D., Rodríguez-García, M.I., and Alché, J.D. (2012). Characterization of profilin polymorphism in pollen with a focus on multifunctionality. *PLoS One*, Vol. 7, No. 2, pp. e30878.

Jonckheere, V., Lambrechts, A., Vandekerckhove, J., and Ampe, C. (1999). Dimerization of profilin II upon binding the (GP5)3 peptide from VASP overcomes the inhibition of actin nucleation by profilin II and thymosin beta4. *FEBS Letter*, Vol. 447, pp. 257–263.

Jockusch, B.M., Murk, K., and Rothkegel, M. (2007). The profile of profilins. *Reviews of physiology, biochemistry and pharmacology*, Vol. 159, pp. 131-149.

Kovar, D.R., Drøbak, B.K., Collings, D.A., and Staiger, C.J. (2001). The characterization of ligand specific maize (*Zea mays*) profilin mutants. *Biochemical Journal*, Vol. 358, pp. 49-57.

Kovar, D.R., Drøbak, B.K., and Staiger, C.J. (2000). Maize profilin isoforms are functionally distinct. *Plant Cell*, Vol. 12, pp. 583-598.

Kandasamy, M.K., McKinney, E.C., and Meagher, R.B. (2002). Plant profilin isovariants are distinctly regulated in vegetative and reproductive tissues. *Cell motility and the cytoskeleton*, Vol. 52, N°. 1, pp. 22-32.

Karakesisoglou, I., Schleicher, M., Gibbon, B.C., and Staiger, C.J. (1996). Plant profilins rescue the aberrant phenotype of profilin-deficient Dictyostelium cells. *Cell motility and the cytoskeleton*, Vol. 34, N°. 1, pp. 36-47.

Levene, H. (1960). Robust tests for equality of variances. In: Ingram Olkin, Harold Hotelling, et al. (Ed.). Stanford University Press, pp 278–292.

López-Torrejón, G., Díaz-Perales, A., Rodríguez, J., Sánchez-Monge, R., Crespo, J.F., Salcedo, G., and Pacios, L.F. (2007). An experimental and modeling-based approach to locate IgE epitopes of plant profilin allergens. *Journal of Allergy and Clinnical Immunology*, Vol. 119, N°. 6, pp. 1481-1488.

Lu, J., and Pollard, T.D. (2001). Profilin binding to poly-L-proline and actin monomers along with ability to catalyze actin nucleotide exchange is required for viability of fission yeast. *Molecular and Cellular Biology*, Vol. 12, pp. 1161–1175.

Marazuela, E.G., Rodríguez, R., Barber, D., Villalba, M., and Batanero, E. (2007). Hypoallergenic mutants of Ole e 1, the major olive pollen allergen, as candidates for allergy vaccines. *Clinnical and experimental allergy*, Vol. 37, N°. 2, pp. 251-60.

Mazzotti, G., Zini, N., Rizzi, E., Rizzoli, R., Galanzi, A., Ognibene, A., Santi, S., Matteucci, A., Martelli, A.M., and Maraldi, N.M. (1995). Immunocytochemical detection of phosphatidylinositol 4,5-biphosphate localization sites within the nucleus. *Journal of Histochemistry and Cytochemistry*, Vol. 43, pp. 181–191.

McDowell, J.M., Huang, S., McKinney, E.C., An, Y.Q., and Meagher, R.B. (1996), Structure and evolution of the actin gene family in *Arabidopsis thaliana*. *Genetics*, Vol. 142, pp. 587–602.

Mehta, C.R., and Patel, N.R. (1983). A network algorithm for performing Fisher's exact test in contingency tables. *Journal of American Statistical Association*, Vol. 78, N°. 382, pp. 427–434.

Morales, S., Jimenez-Lopez, J.C., Castro, A.J., Rodríguez-García, M.I., and Alché, J.D. (2008). Olive pollen profilin (Ole e 2 allergen) co-localizes with highly active areas of the actin cytoskeleton and is released to the culture medium during in vitro pollen germination. *Journal of Microscopy-Oxford*, Vol. 231, No. 2, pp. 332-341.

Neidt, E.M., Scott, B.J., and Kovar, D.R. (2009). Formin differentially utilizes profilin isoforms to rapidly assemble actin filaments. *Journal of Biological Chemistry*, Vol. 284, pp. 673–684.

Piboonpocanun, S., Malainual, N., Jirapongsananuruk, O., Vichyanond, P., and Thomas, W.R. (2006). Genetic polymorphisms of major house dust mite allergens. *Clinnical and experimental allergy*, Vol. 36, pp. 510-516.

Psaradellis, T., Kao, N.L, and Babich, M. (2000). Recombinant Zea mays profilin forms multimers with pan-allergenic potential. *Allergology International*, Vol. 49, pp. 27–35.

Radauer, C., Willerroider, M., Fuchs, H., Hoffmann-Sommergruber, K., Thalhamer, J., Ferreira, F., and Scheiner, O. & Breiteneder H. (2006). Cross-reactive and species-specific immunoglobulin E epitopes of plant profilins: an experimental and structure-based analysis. *Clinnical and experimental allergy*, Vol. 36, N. 7, pp. 920-929.

Rando, O.J., Zhao, K., and Crabtree, G.R. (2000). Searching for a function for nuclear actin. *Trends in Cell Biology*, Vol. 10, pp. 92-97.

Schmidt von Braun, S., and Schleiff, E. (2008). The chloroplast outer membrane protein Chup1 interacts with actin and profilin. *Planta*, Vol. 227, N°. 5, pp. 1151-1159.

Seong, S.Y., and Matzinger, P. (2004). Hydrophobicity: an ancient damage-associated molecular pattern that initiates innate immune responses. *Nature Immunology*, Vol. 4, N°. 6, pp. 469-478.

Shapiro, S.S., and Wilk, M.B. (1965). An analysis of variance for normality (complete samples). *Biometrika*, Vol. 52, pp. 591–611.

Thorn, K.S., Christensen, H.E., Shigeta, R., Huddler, D., Lindberg, U., Chua, N.H., and Schutt, C.E. (1997). The crystal structure of a major allergen from plants. *Structure*, Vol. 5, pp. 19-32.

Valenta, R., Ball, T., Vrtala, S., Duchêne, M., Kraft, D., and Scheiner, O. (1994). cDNA cloning and expression of timothy grass (Phleum pratense) pollen profilin in Escherichia coli: comparison with birch pollen profilin. *Biochemical and biophysical research communications*, Vol. 199, N. 1, pp. 106-118.

Valenta, R., Duchêne, M., Pettenburger, K., Sillaber, C., Valent, P., Bettelheim, P., Breitenbach, M., and Rumpold, H., Kraft, D., and Scheiner, O. (1991). Identification of profilin as a novel pollen allergen; IgE autoreactivity in sensitized individuals. *Science*, Vol. 253, pp. 557-560.

Vallverdu, A., Asturias, J.A., Arilla, M.C., Gomez-Bayon, N., Martinez, A., and Martinez, J., and Palacios R. (1998). Characterization of recombinant Mercurialis annua major allergen Mer a 1 (profilin). *Journal of Allergy and Clinnical Immunology*, Vol. 101, N°. 3, pp. 363–370.

Valster, A.H., Vidali, L., and Hepler, P.K. (2003). Nuclear localization of profilin during the cell cycle in *Tradescantia virginiana* stamen hair cells. *Protoplasma*, Vol. 222, pp. 85–95.

van Ree, R. (2004). Clinical importance of cross-reactivity in food allergy. *Current Opinion in Allergy and Clinnical Immunology*, Vol. 4, N°. 3, pp. 235-240.

Vidali, L., and Hepler, P.K. (1997). Characterization and localization of profilin in pollen grains and tubes of Lilium longiflorum. *Cell motility and the cytoskeleton*, Vol. 36, N°. 4, pp. 323-338.

Vidali, L., Pérez, H.E., Valdés López, V., Noguez, R., Zamudio, F., and Sánchez, F. (1995). Purification, characterization, and cDNA cloning of profilin from Phaseolus vulgaris. *Plant physiology*, Vol. 108, N°. 1, pp. 115-123.

von Witsch, M., Baluška, F., Staiger, C.J., and Volkmann, D. (1998). Profilin is associated with the plasma membrane in microspores and pollen. *European Journal of Cell Biology*, Vol. 77, N°. 4, pp. 303-312.

Yoneda, Y. (1997). How proteins are transported from cytoplasm to the nucleus. *Journal of Biochemistry*, Vol. 121, pp. 811-817.

Chapter 6

Efficacy of Flavonoids for Patients with Japanese Cedar Pollinosis

Toshio Tanaka

Additional information is available at the end of the chapter

http://dx.doi.org/10.5772/45882

1. Introduction

The worldwide prevalence of allergic diseases such as asthma, atopic dermatitis and allergic rhinitis has increased during the last two decades (Holgate, 1999; Eder et al., 2006). Allergic rhinitis now affects 400-500 million people worldwide (Greiner et al., 2011; Ozdoganoglu & Songu, 2012) and adversely affects social life, school performance, and work productivity (Bousquet et al., 2001). The first case of Japanese cedar pollinosis in Japan was reported in the mid-1960s (Horiguchi & Saito, 1964), but now half of the Japanese population have become sensitized to Japanese cedar pollens and 24-29% of the population is suffering from the disease (Kaneko et al., 2005), so that Japanese cedar pollinosis is now rated as one of the most common diseases in Japan (Okamoto et al., 2009). The complicated interaction between genetic and environmental factors is thought to cause the development of allergic diseases. Many genetic loci related to atopy, a genetic tendency to produce immunoglobulin E (IgE) in response to environmental allergens, have been identified through genome-wide association studies (Grammatikos, 2008). However, changes in the environment have made a more significant contribution than genetic factors to the recent increase in the prevalence of allergic diseases (Nolte et al., 2001; Ho, 2010), since it seems unlikely that genes would have changed during the last two decades. Dietary change has been proposed as one of the environmental factors responsible for the increasing prevalence or the worsening symptoms of allergic diseases (Devereux & Seaton, 2005; Devereux, 2006; Kozyrskyj et al., 2011; Nurmatov et al., 2011; Allan & Devereux, 2011). Indeed foods include both allergy-promoting and anti-allergic nutrients (McKeever & Britton, 2004), and flavonoids, which are plant secondary metabolites, can have powerful antioxidant, anti-allergic and immune-modulating effects (Hollman & Katan, 1999; Middleton et al., 2000; Manach et al., 2004). This review article introduces the anti-allergic properties and efficacy of flavonoids for patients with Japanese cedar pollinosis and discusses the possibility that an appropriate intake of flavonoids may constitute an effective complementary and alternative medicine as well as a preventative strategy for allergic diseases.

2. Flavonoids possess anti-allergic activity

In the mid-1990s we evaluated the clinical efficacy of one kind of traditional vegetarian diet on adult patients with severely to moderately active atopic dermatitis. After a two-month treatment period, the severity of dermatitis had decreased from 49.9 to 27.4 based on the SCORAD index, a score of atopic dermatitis severity, in association with a reduction in the number of peripheral blood eosinophils and the amount of urinary secretion of 8-hydroxy-2′-deoxyguanosine, a marker of oxidative DNA damage (Kouda et al., 2000; Tanaka et al., 2001). What factor(s) led to this amelioration of dermatitis remained unknown but subsequently it was found that one of the characteristics of the remedy was a high daily intake of flavonoids.

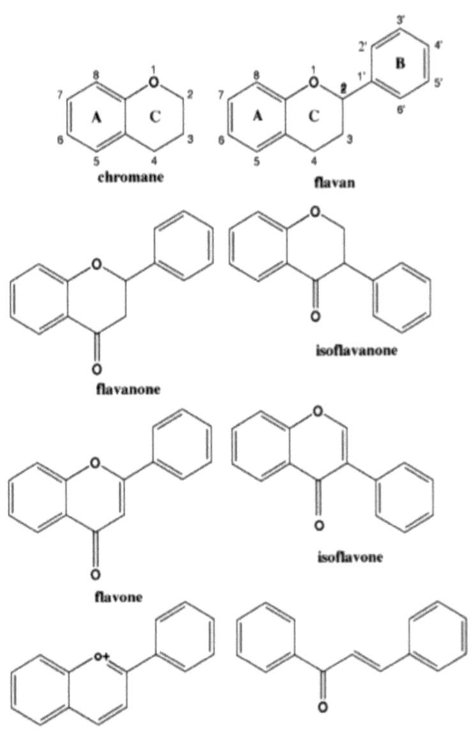

Figure 1. Structures of basic flavonoid skeletons

Flavonoids are comprised of a large group of low-molecular-weight polyphenolic secondary plant metabolites that are found in fruit, vegetables, cereals and beverages, and thus are common substances in the daily diet (Hollman & Katan, 1999; Middleton et al., 2000). Based on their skeleton, flavonoids are classified into eight groups: flavans, flavanones, isoflavanones, flavones, isoflavones, anthocyanidins, chalcones and flavonolignans (Fig. 1).

Flavonols constitute a separate class of flavonoids that possess the 3-hydroxyflavone backbone. Typical flavonoids such as quercetin, kaempferol, fisetin and myricetin belong to flavonols while luteolin and apigenin are classified as flavones. Flavonoids have been found to exert several biological activities including antioxidant, anti-bacterial and anti-viral activities, and to have anti-inflammatory, anti-angionic, analgestic, hepatoprotective, cytostatic, apoptotic, estrogenic or anti-estrogenic and immune-modulating effects as well as anti-allergic properties (Harborne & Williams, 2000; Williams & Grayer, 2004; Chirumbolo, 2010; Visioli et al., 2011; Calderon-Montano et al., 2011; Russo et al., 2012). As a result, considerable interest has been paid to the role of flavonoids in the prevention of chronic diseases, including cardiovascular diseases, cancers, type 2 diabetes, neurodegenerative diseases, osteoporosis and allergic diseases (Sealbert et al., 2005).

Mast cells and basophils expressing the high-affinity IgE receptor (FcεRI) play an important role in allergic inflammation by releasing chemical mediators such as histamine and cyteinyl leukotrienes, cytokines and chemokines (Stone et al., 2010). As for the anti-allergic activities of flavonoids, Fewtress and Gomperts first identified the inhibition by flavones of transport ATPase in histamine secretion from rat mast cells (Fewtrell & Gomperts, 1997). Fisetin, quercetin, myricetin and kaempferol were found to inhibit histamine release while morin and rutin showed little effect. Subsequently, quercetin was reported to inhibit histamine release by allergen-stimulated human basophils (Middleton et al., 1981; Middleton & Kandaswami, 1992). Flavonoids such as apigenin, luteolin, 3,6-dihydroxy flavones, fisetin, kaempferol, quercetin, and myricetin, all with IC_{50} values of less than 10 μM, were found to inhibit hexosaminidase release from rat mast cells (Cheong et al., 1998). In addition, flavonoids have also been shown to suppress cysteinyl leukotriene synthesis through inhibition of phospholipase A_2 and 5-lipoxygenase (Lee et al., 1982; Yoshimoto et al., 1983). As for the suppressive effect of flavonoids on cytokine expression, Kimata et al were the first to report that luteolin, quercetin and baicalein inhibited the secretion of granulocyte macrophage-colony stimulating factor by human cultured mast cells in response to cross-linkage of FcεRI (Kimata et al., 2000a) and subsequently showed that these compounds also inhibited IgE-mediated tumor necrosis factor (TNF)-α and interleukin (IL)-6 production by bone marrow-derived cultured murine mast cells (Kimata et al., 2000b). These findings thus indicate that flavonoids are inhibitors of chemical mediator release and cytokine production by mast cells and basophils. One of the characteristic features of allergic diseases is overproduction of IgE in response to environmental allergens. The differentiation of B cells into IgE-producing cells requires both the interaction of the CD40 ligand with CD40 and the action of IL-4 or IL-13 on B cells (Rosenwasser, 2011), which are provided with these signals by Th2 cells, basophils and mast cells (Gauchat et al., 1993). Basophils were then used to examine the effects of flavonoids on IL-4, IL-13 and CD40 ligand expression. It was found that fisetin suppressed in a dose-dependent fashion both IL-4 and IL-13 synthesis by allergen- or anti-IgE antibody-stimulated peripheral blood basophils and that the IC_{50} value of fisetin for inhibition of IL-4 synthesis was 5.8 μM (Higa et al., 2003; Hirano et al., 2004). Fisetin also inhibited IL-4, IL-5 and IL-13 production by KU812 cells, a basophilic cell line, in response to the calcium ionophore, A23187 plus phorbol myristate acetate (PMA), but the suppressive effect of fisetin on IL-6, IL-8 and IL-1β synthesis was relatively weak (Higa et al., 2003). In order to determine the basic structure of the flavonoids that accounts for their inhibition of IL-4 production and to identify more active compounds, 45 kinds of flavones, flavonols and their related compounds were screened (Hirano et al., 2004; Kawai et al., 2007).

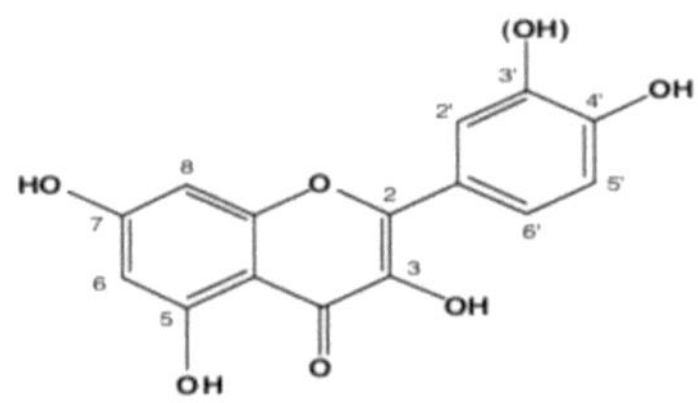

(Each OH for 3 or 5 position)

	3	5	6	7	8	2'	3'	4'	5'	6'	IC_{50} (μM)
Luteolin	H	OH	H	OH	H	H	OH	OH	H	H	2.7
Apigenin	H	OH	H	OH	H	H	H	OH	H	H	3.1
Fisetin	OH	H	H	OH	H	H	OH	OH	H	H	5.8
Compound 6	H	OH	H	H	H	H	OH	OH	OH	H	11.4
Scutellarein	H	OH	OH	OH	H	H	H	OH	H	H	14.0
Kaempferol	OH	OH	H	OH	H	H	H	OH	H	H	15.7
Quercetin	OH	OH	H	OH	H	H	OH	OH	H	H	18.8
7-Hydroxyflavone	H	H	H	OH	H	H	H	H	H	H	26.5
Myricetin	OH	OH	H	OH	H	H	OH	OH	OH	H	>30
Galangin	OH	OH	H	OH	H	H	H	H	H	H	>30
Baicalein	H	OH	OH	OH	H	H	H	H	H	H	>30

Figure 2. Basic structure of flavonoids for inhibitory activity of IL-4 synthesis by basophils

Luteolin, apigenin and fisetin were found to be the strongest inhibitors with an IC_{50} value of 2.7-5.8 μM (Fig. 2). Quercetin and kaempferol are representative of flavonoids associated with a substantial daily intake and had an intermediate inhibitory effect on IL-4 synthesis with an IC_{50} value of 15.7-18.8 μM, but myricetin showed no such effect. These analyses of structure-activity relationships revealed the fundamental structure required for the action. For maximal effect, hydroxylation in positions 7 and 4' is essential while the presence of OH in either position 3 or 5 is also required. In addition, luteolin, apigenin and fisetin were found to suppress CD40 ligand expression by activated basophils and KU812 cells in a dose-dependent manner, whereas myricetin even at 30 μM did not have such an effect (Hirano et al., 2006). These inhibitory properties indicate that flavonoids such as luteolin, apigenin and fisetin are natural IgE inhibitors.

The aryl hydrocarbon receptor (AhR) is a ligand-activated transcriptional factor that mediates the toxic and biological actions of many aromatic environmental pollutants such as dioxins (Connor & Aylward, 2006). An AhR-based in vitro bioassay for the dioxin [2,3,7,8-tetrachlorodibenzo-*p*-dioxin (TCDD)] revealed that the flavonoids, apigenin, luteolin, baicalein, quercetin, kaempferol and myricetin had noticeable inhibitory effects on AhR activation with an EC_{70} value (equal to 70% of the maximal response to TCDD) of 1.9-5.1 μM, while marked AhR activation was displayed by daidzein, resveratrol, naringenin and baicalein at higher concentrations (Amakura et al., 2008). Moreover, it has recently been shown that AhR is a regulator of differentiation of naïve CD4 positive T cells into effector T cell subsets (Marshall & Kerkvliet, 2010), suggesting that flavonoids modulate immune functions through their binding to AhR.

3. The relationship between flavonoid intake and the prevalence, incidence or severity of allergic diseases

As mentioned previously, flavonoids are contained in vegetables, fruit, cereals and beverages. Epidemiological studies have reported that a high intake of fresh fruit and vegetables may provide protection against asthma (La Vecchia et al., 1998; Butland et al., 1999). The Mediterranean diet, which has high antioxidant content because of the preponderance of fruit, vegetables, legumes, nuts and wholegrain cereals, has been associated with a reduced likelihood of asthma, wheezing and allergic rhinitis in cross-sectional studies of children (Chatzi et al., 2007; Garcia-Marcos et al., 2007; Tamay et al., 2007; De Batlle et al., 2008; Castro-Rodriguez et al., 2008). Shaheen et al reported that the results of a population-based case-control study of 607 cases and 864 controls in South London indicated that apple consumption and red wine intake were negatively associated with, respectively, asthma prevalence and severity, perhaps due to the protective effect of flavonoids (Shaheen et al., 2001), while the follow-up study made it clear that dietary intake of catechins, flavonols and flavones was not significantly associated with asthma prevalence and severity (Garcia et al., 2005). A cohort epidemiological study of 10,054 adults in Finland regarding the association between flavonoid intake and risk of several chronic diseases found that asthma incidence was lower for higher quercetin, naringenin, and hesperetin intakes (Knekt et al., 2002).

A study of 1,253 five-year-old children reported that maternal apple intake during their mothers' pregnancy was associated with beneficial results for ever wheeze, ever asthma and doctor-confirmed asthma (Willers et al., 2007). The Irish Lifeways Cross-Generation Cohort Study determined an association between high maternal fruit and vegetable intake during pregnancy and reduced likelihood of asthma in 632 three-year-old children (Fitzsimon et al., 2007). A third cohort study also demonstrated that wheeze and atopic sensitization in 460 children aged 6-7 years was less frequent if their mothers had followed a Mediterranean diet during pregnancy (Chatzi et al., 2008). Although there have been few reports of case-control or longitudinal studies examining direct associations between flavonoid intake and the prevalence or incidence of allergic diseases, the findings of the epidemiological studies mentioned here suggest that higher flavonoid intake is beneficial for protection against allergic diseases.

4. Efficacy of flavonoids in allergic models

The anti-allergic characteristics of flavonoids observed *in vitro* led to a study using NC/Nga mice to test whether intake of flavonoids might be effective for the prevention or the amelioration of allergic symptoms. NC/Nga mice spontaneously develop severe eczema, scratching behaviour and serum IgE elevation with aging under nonspecific pathogen-free conditions (Matsuda et al., 1997). To determine the preventive effect of flavonoids, the mice were orally given astragalin, kaempferol 3'glucoside (1.5 mg/kg), a major ingredient of flavonoid in persimmon leaf tea, or a control diet. Development of dermatitis with aging was observed in the control group and the severity of dermatitis was scored for evaluation. Oral intake of astragalin markedly prevented the appearance of the dermal symptoms, scratching behaviour and serum IgE elevation (Kotani et al., 2000). Moreover, when astragalin was administered to NC/Nga mice after the appearance of dermatitis, it significantly diminished its severity (Matsumoto et al., 2002). It was subsequently demonstrated with this mouse model that administration of extracts from petals of *Impatiens balsamina* L., which contains flavonoids such as kaempferol 3-rutinoside and 2-hydroxy-1,4-naphthoquinone as active gradients (Oku & Ishiguro, 2001), of apigenin (Yano et al., 2009), or of baicalein (Yun et al., 2010) suppressed skin lesions. In an asthmatic mouse model sensitized with ovalbumin (OVA), it was demonstrated that oral administration of luteolin, even as little as 0.1 mg/kg, led to a significant suppression of bronchial hyperreactivity and bronchoconstriction (Das et al., 2003). It was also found that nobiletin, a polymethoxyflavonoid, when given intraperitoneally to OVA-sensitized rats at a dose of 1.5 or 5 mg/kg, reduced OVA-induced increases in eosinophils and eotaxin expression (Wu et al., 2006). In subsequent investigations, flavonoids such as quercetin, isoquercitrin, rutin, 3-*O*-methylquercetin 5,7,3',4'-*O*-tetraacetate, narirutin, apigenin, luteolin, sulfuretin, hesperdin, fisetin and kaempferol have been shown to suppress responses in various types of allergic animals (Makino et al., 2001; Fernandez et al., 2005; Rogerio et al., 2007; Jung et al., 2007; Jiang et al., 2007; Funaguchi et al., 2007; Yano et al., 2007; Cruz et al., 2008; Park et al., 2009; Choi et al., 2009; Li et al., 2010; Leemans et al., 2010; Shishebor et al., 2010; Song et al., 2010; Kim et al., 2011; Wu et al., 2011; Gong et al., 2012).

5. Efficacy of flavonoids for patients with allergic rhinitis

The aforementioned findings regarding the *in vitro* and *in vivo* anti-allergic properties of flavonoids strongly support the notion that an appropriate intake of flavonoids may constitute a complementary and alternative medicine and/or a preventive strategy for allergic diseases (Tanaka et al., 2003; Tanaka et al., 2004; Kawai et al., 2007; Tanaka et al., 2011; Singh et al., 2011). Indeed, the results of previous clinical trials using flavonoid extracts suggest that flavonoids have beneficial effects on allergic rhinitis (Takano et al., 2004; Kishi et al., 2005; Enomoto et al., 2006; Segawa et al., 2007; Yoshimura et al., 2007). The extracts examined were *Perilla frutescens* enriched with rosmarinic acid, apple polyphenols including procyanidins, or apple condensed tannin, catechin, epicatechin, phlorizin, and chlorogenic acid, hop water extract including quercetin and kaempferol glycosides, and tomato extract including mainly naringenin chalcone. However, the direct effect of flavonoids on allergic symptoms has remained unknown.

Enzymatically modified isoquercitrin (EMIQ) is a quercetin glycoside that consists of isoquercitrin and its maltooligosaccharides, and is manufactured from rutin through an enzymatic modification (Fig. 3) (Salim et al., 2004), which markedly enhances the absorption rate through the intestine.

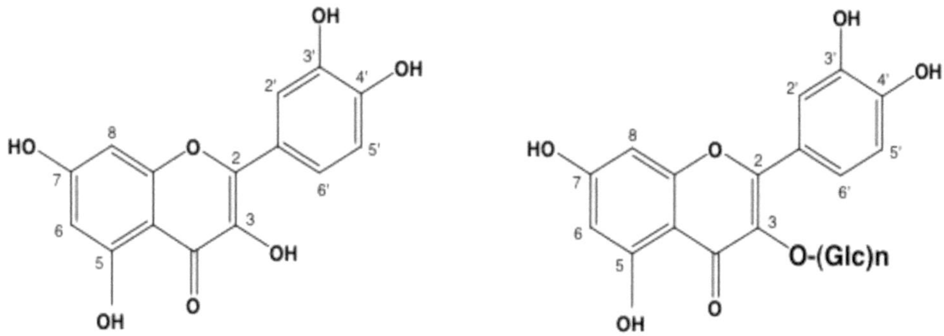

Quercetin

Enzymatically modified isoquercitrin EMIQ (n=1~8)

Figure 3. Enzymatically modified isoquercitrin is a quercetin glycoside.

This flavonoid is approved as a food additive in Japan and is used as an antioxidant for various commercially available food products such as beverages. Tests were performed in 2007, 2008 and 2009 to determine whether intake of EMIQ was effective for Japanese cedar pollinosis (Kawai et al., 2009; Hirano et al., 2009). Japanese cedar pollinosis is defined as an immunological response modulated by IgE and a seasonal (intermittent) allergic rhinoconjunctivitis caused by Japanese cedar pollen, characterized by nasal symptoms such as sneezing, rhinorrhea and nasal congestion and by ocular symptoms such as lacrimation, ocular itching and congestion (Okamoto et al., 2009).

In a parallel-group, double-blind, placebo-controlled study, volunteers with Japanese cedar pollinosis took two capsules of 50 mg EMIQ or a placebo daily for 8 weeks during the pollen season. Severity of subjective symptoms was evaluated by a scoring system (Baba et al, 2002) with some modifications. The study in 2007 began after the pollen had dispersed and thus aimed at examining the therapeutic effect of EMIQ. During the entire study period, ocular symptom+medication and ocular symptom scores for the EMIQ group were significantly lower than those for the placebo group (Fig. 4), while symptom+medication and symptom scores were significantly reduced at week 4-5 compared to those for the placebo group (Kawai et al., 2009).

To examine the preventive effect of EMIQ on symptoms of pollinosis the next study in 2008 began 3 weeks before the first day of pollen dispersion. Ocular symptom+medication and ocular symptom scores were also significantly suppressed during the entire period and symptom+medication and symptom scores were also reduced at week 5-6 (Fig. 5) (Hirano et al., 2009).

Although these two studies did not show a statistically significant ameliorative effect on nasal symptoms, the 2009 study using 200 mg/day of EMIQ for 4 weeks clearly demonstrated efficacy of EMIQ for reducing nasal symptoms (Fig. 6).

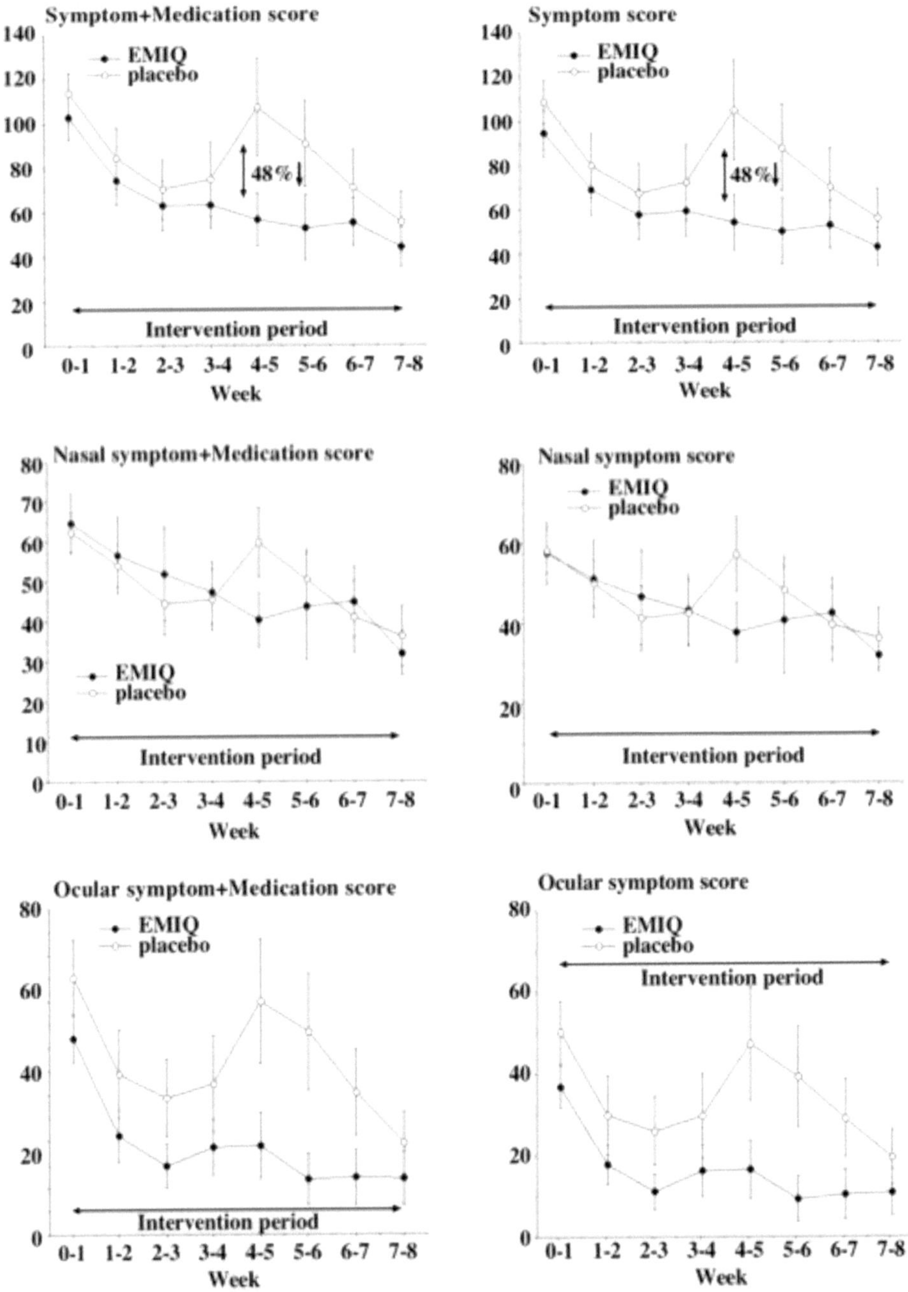

Figure 4. Efficacy of EMIQ on allergic symptoms caused by Japanese cedar pollinosis in 2007. The ameliorative effect was evaluated by total symptom (nasal+ocular symptom)+medication, total symptom, nasal symptom (sneezing, rhinorrhea and nasal obstruction)+medication, nasal symptom, ocular symptom (ocular itching, lacrimation and ocular congestion)+medication and ocular symptom scores.

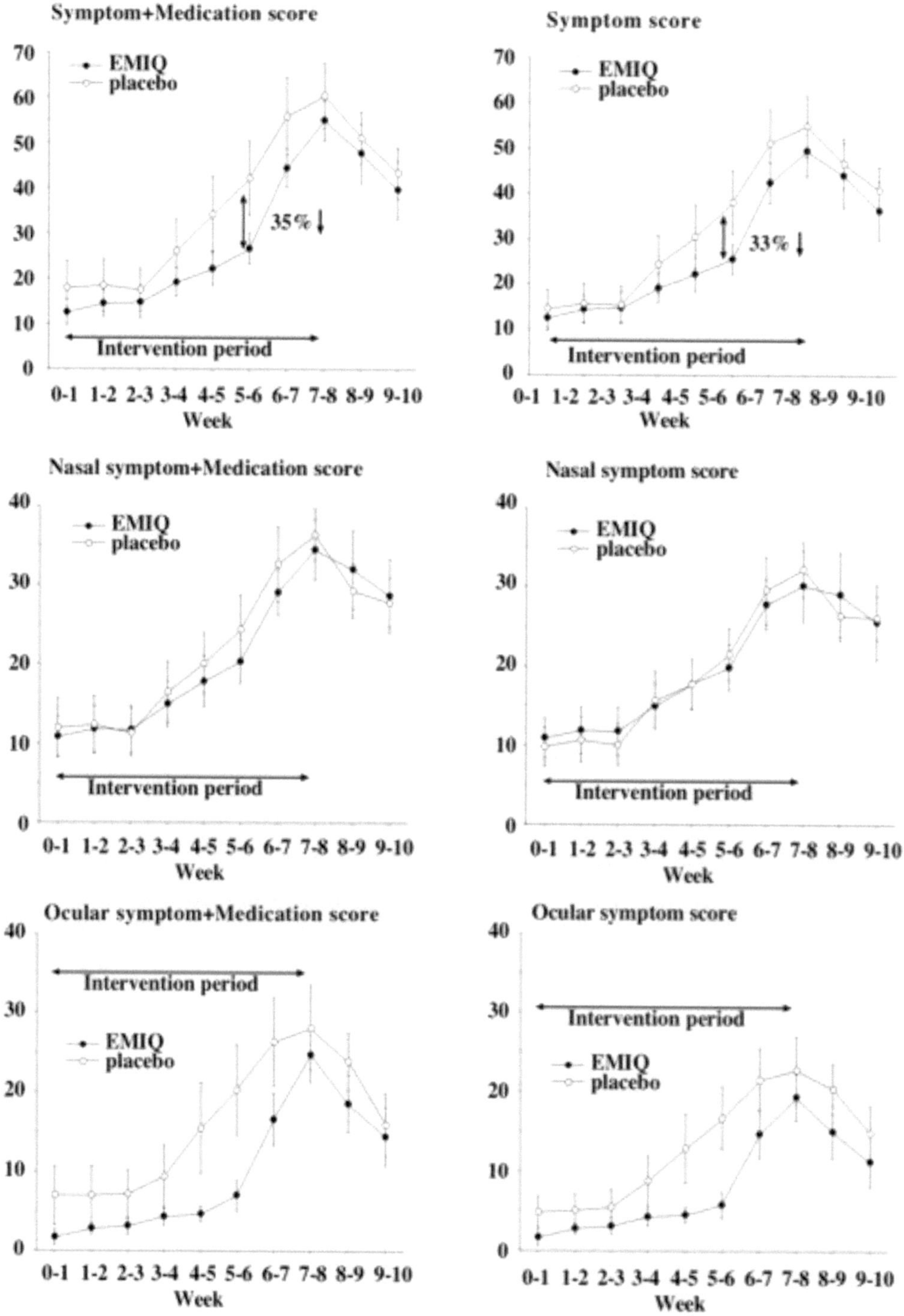

Figure 5. Efficacy of EMIQ on allergic symptoms caused by Japanese cedar pollinosis in 2008.

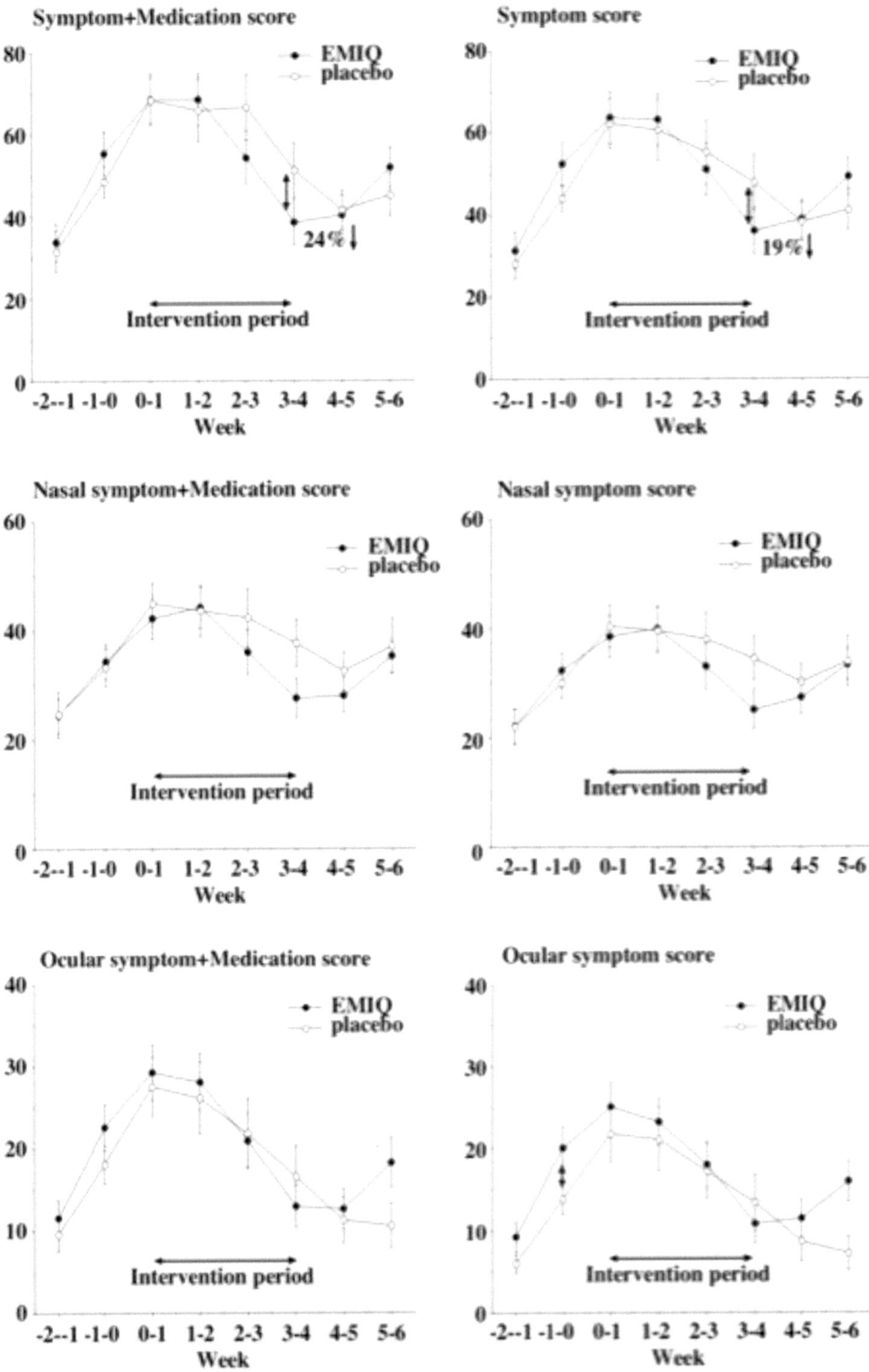

Figure 6. Efficacy of EMIQ on allergic symptoms caused by Japanese cedar pollinosis in 2009.

Moreover, a recent study showed the beneficial action of silymarin on allergic rhinitis symptoms (Bakshaee et al., 2011), and clinical trials of pycnogenol, derived from the bark of the European coastal pine tree, including proanthocyanidines (Wilson et al., 2010), and of benifuuki green tea containing *O*-methylated catechin (Maeda-Yamamoto et al., 2009) demonstrated their ameliorative effects on seasonal allergic rhinitis symptoms.

6. Flavonoid daily intake and content of foods

Clinical trials of EMIQ involving patients with Japanese cedar pollinosis demonstrated that a daily intake of 100-200 mg of EMIQ is effective for the amelioration of symptoms. 100 mg of EMIQ, a glycosylated quercetin, is equivalent to 34 mg of quercetin. Results for the daily intake of flavonols plus flavones calculated in terms of the amounts of quercetin, kaempferol and myricetin, and, in some studies, with the addition of luteolin, apigenin and fisetin, have been reported in several countries (Tanaka et al., 2004). The total amount of these flavonoids varied from 2.6 to 68.2 mg/day in the European Union, USA and Japan. The major flavonoid was quercetin, ranging from 14 to 100% of the total amount of flavonoids, followed by kaempferol and myricetin with an average intake of 0.1 to 5.9 mg/day. An amount of 34 mg/day of quercetin is therefore tolerable and indeed there were no adverse events in the clinical trials. Recently, the U.S. Department of Agriculture (USDA) database for the flavonoid content of selected foods was published (USDA database, release 3, 2011). The database contains values for 500 food items and for 28 predominant monomeric dietary flavonoids that include quercetin, kaempferol, myricetin, apigenin and luteolin. It should be pointed out that most of the compounds in food are present in glycosylated forms, but this database converted the glycoside values into aglycone forms using conversion factors based on the molecular weight of the specific compounds to make data consistent across the database. EuroFIR-BASIS (European Food Information Resource - Bioactive Substances in Food Information System) is another database currently developed for bioactives that covers original content values for various polyphenols in plant-based foods (Gry et al., 2007). The more recently published Phenol-Explorer database includes content data for 502 polyphenols, flavonoids, phenolic acids, lignans, and stilbenes (Neveu et al., 2010; database URL: http://www.phenol-explorer.eu/; Perez-Jimenez et al., 2010). Over 60,000 composition data published since 1969 have been systemically collected, evaluated, and stored in this database and it contains information on glycosides and esters, whereas the USDA database pertains to data on aglycones. The Phenol-Explorer database was used to examine the intake of all individual polyphenols by a total of middle-aged 4,942 men and women in France (Perez-Jimenez et al., 2011). Mean total intake of flavonoids including proanthocyanidins, catechins, anthocyanins, flavonols, flavones, flavanones, theaflavins and dihydroflavonols was estimated at 506 mg/day, with nonalcoholic beverages, fruit, alcoholic beverages, cocoa products, vegetables and cereals contributing 114, 172, 73, 90, 26 and 28 mg/day, respectively. Mean total intake of flavonols and flavones was 51 and 33 mg/day, which is equivalent to 34 and 18 mg/day of aglycones, respectively. The findings obtained with these databases are sure to make a significant contribution to the development of dietary treatment for allergic rhinitis.

7. Conclusion

Allergy, a common disease worldwide, is the subject of growing concern because of its increasing rate of prevalence (Holgate, 1999; Eder et al, 2006). It has been suggested that dietary changes may contribute to this increase (McKeever & Britton, 2004; Devereux & Seaton, 2005; Devereux, 2006; Kozyrskyj et al., 2011; Nurmatov et al., 2011; Allan & Devereux, 2011). Flavonoids have antioxidant, anti-allergic and immune-modulating properties and recent clinical trials have shown their beneficial effect on allergic rhinitis. Several extensive databases for the flavonoid content of major vegetables, fruit, cereals and beverages can thus be expected to contribute to the dietary management of allergic rhinitis. Whether an appropriate intake of flavonoids can ameliorate respiratory or dermal allergic symptoms and prevent the onset of allergic diseases thus constitutes an important issue for future studies.

Author details

Toshio Tanaka
Department of Respiratory Medicine, Allergy and Rheumatic Diseases,
Department of Clinical Application of Biologics, Osaka University Graduate School of Medicine, and
Department of Immunopathology, WPI Immunology Frontier Research Center,
Osaka University, Osaka, Japan

Acknowledgement

The author thanks Dr. Mari Kawai, Dr. Toru Hirano, Dr. Shinji Higa, Ms. Mihoko Koyanagi, Ms. Tomoko Kai, Mr. Ryosuke Shimizu, Dr. Masamitsu Moriwaki, Dr. Yukio Suzuki, and Dr. Satoshi Ogino as collaborators for the clinical studies.

8. References

Allan, K. & Devereux, G. (2011). Diet and asthma: nutrition implications from prevention to treatment. *Journal of the American Dietetic Association*, Vol.111, No.2, (February 2011), pp. 258-268.

Amakura, Y.; Tsutsumi, T.; Sasaki, K.; Nakamura, M.; Yoshida, T. & Maitani, T. (2008). Influence of food polyphenols on aryl hydrocarbon receptor-signaling pathway estimated by in vitro bioassay. *Phytochemistry*, Vol.69, No.18, (December 2008), pp. 3117-3130.

Baba, K.; Konno, A. & Takenaka, H. (2002). Epidemiology. *in* Okuda, M. (ed.), *Guidelines for treatment of nasal allergy-perennial rhinitis and pollinosis.* Life Science Publishing, Tokyo, 2002, pp. 8-11.

Bakhshaee, M.; Jabbari, F.; Hoseini, S.; Farid, R.; Sadeghian, M.H.; Rajati, M.; Mohamadpoor, A.H.; Movahhed, R. & Zamani, M.A. (2011). Effect of silymarin in the treatment of allergic rhinitis. *Otolaryngology-Head and Neck Surgery*, Vol.145, No.6, (December 2011), pp. 904-909.

Bousquet, J.; Van Cauwenberge, P. & Khaltaev, N.; Aria Workshop Group: World Health Organization. (2001). Allergic rhinitis and its impact on asthma. *Journal of Allergy and Clinical Immunology*, Vol.108(5 Suppl), (November 2001), pp. S147-334.

Butland, B.K.; Strachan, D.P. & Anderson, H.R. (1999). Fresh fruit intake and asthma symptoms in young British adults: confounding or effect modification by smoking? *European Respiratory Journal*, Vol.13, No.4, (April 1999), pp. 744-750.

Calderon-Montano, J.M.; Burgos-Moron, E.; Perez-Guerrero, C. & Lopez-Lazaro, M. (2011). A review on the dietary flavonoid kaempferol. *Mini-Reviews in Medicinal Chemistry*, Vol.11, No.4, (April 2011), pp. 298-344.

Castro-Rodriguez, J.A.; Garcia-Marcos, L.; Alfonseda Rojas, J.D.; Valverde-Molina, J. & Sanchez-Solis, M. (2008). Mediterranean diet as a protective factor for wheezing in preschool children. *The Journal of Pediatrics*, Vol.152, No.6, (June 2008), pp. 823-828.

Chatzi, L.; Apostolaki, G.; Bibakis, I.; Skypala, I.; Bibaki-Liakou, V.; Tzanakis, N.; Kogevinas, M. & Cullinan, P. (2007). Protective effect of fruits, vegetables and the Mediterranean diet on asthma and allegies among children in Crete. *Thorax*, Vol.62, No.8, (August 2007), pp. 677-683.

Chatzi, L.; Torrent, M.; Romieu, I.; Garcia-Esteban, R.; Ferrer, C.; Vioque, J.; Kogevinas, M. & Sunyer, J. (2008). Mediterranean diet in pregnancy is protective for wheeze and atopy in childhood. *Thorax*, Vol.63, No.6, (June 2008), pp. 507-513.

Cheong, H.; Ryu, S.Y.; Oak, M.H.; Cheon, S.H.; Yoo, G.S. & Kim, K.M. (1998). Studies of structure activity relationship of flavonoids for the anti-allergic actions. *Archives of Pharmacal Research*, Vol.21, No.4, (August 1998), pp. 478-480.

Chirumbolo, S. (2010). The role of quercetin, flavonols and flavones in modulating inflammatory cell function. *Inflammatory & Allergy Drug Targets*, Vol.9, No.4, (September 2010), pp. 263-285.

Choi, J.R.; Lee, C.M.; Jung, I.D.; Lee, J.S.; Jeong, Y.I.; Chang, J.H.; Park, H.J.; Choi, I.W.; Kim, J.S.; Shin, Y.K.; Park, S.N. & Park, Y.M. (2009). Apigenin protects ovalbumin-induced asthma through the regulation of GATA-3 gene. *International Immunopharmacology*, Vol.9, No.7-8, (July 2009), pp. 918-924.

Connor, K.T. & Aylward, L.L. (2006). Human response to dioxin: aryl hydrocarbon receptor (AhR) molecular structure, function, and dose-response data for enzyme induction indicate an impaired human AhR. *Journal of Toxicology and Environmental Health, Part B: Critical Reviews*, Vol.9, No.2, (December 2006), pp. 147-171.

Cruz, E.A.; Da-Silva, S.A.; Muzitano, M.F.; Silva, P.M.; Costa, S.S. & Rossi-Bergmann, B. (2008). Immunomodulatory pretreatment with *Kalanchoe pinnata* extract and its quercitrin flavonoid effectively protects mice against fatal anaphylactic shock. *International Immunopharmacology*, Vol.8, No.12, (December 2008), pp. 1616-1621.

Das, M.; Ram, A. & Ghosh, B. (2003). Luteolin alleviates bronchoconstriction and airway hyperreactivity in ovalbumin sensitized mice. *Inflammation Research*, Vol.52, No.3, (March 2003), pp. 101-106.

De Batlle, J.; Garcia-Aymerich, J.; Barraza-Villarreal, A.; Anto, J.M. & Romieu, I. (2008). Mediterranean diet is associated with reduced asthma and rhinitis in Mexican children. *Allergy*, Vol.63, No.10, (October 2008), pp. 1310-1316.

Devereux, G. & Seaton, A. (2005). Diet as a risk factor for atopy and asthma. *Journal of Allergy and Clinical Immunology*, Vol.115, No.6, (June 2005), pp. 1109-1117.

Devereux, G. (2006). The increase in the prevalence of asthma and allergy: food for thought. *Nature Reviews Immunology*, Vol.6, No.11, (November 2006), pp. 869-874.

Eder, W.; Ege, M.J. & von Mutius, E. (2006). The asthma epidemic. *The New England Journal of Medicine*, Vol.355, No.21, (November 2006), pp. 2226-2235.

Enomoto, T.; Nagasako-Akazome, Y.; Kanda, T.; Ikeda, M. & Dake, T. (2006). Clinical effects of apple polyphenols on persistent allergic rhinitis: a randomized double-blind placebo-controlled parallel arm study. *Journal of Investigational Allergolology and Clinical Immunology*, Vol.16, No.5, (October 2006), pp. 283-289.

Fernandez, J.; Reyes, R.; Ponce, H.; Oropeza, M.; Vancalsteren, M.R.; Jankowski, C. & Campos, M.G. (2005). Isoquercitrin from Argemone platyceras inhibits carbachol and leukotriene D4-induced contraction in guinea-pig airways. *European Journal of Pharmacology*, Vol.522, No.1-3, (October 2005), pp. 108-115.

Fewtrell, C.M. & Gomperts, B.D. (1997). Effect of flavone inhibitors on transport ATPases on histamine secretion from rat mast cells. *Nature*, Vol.265, No.5595, (February 1997), pp. 635-636.

Fitzsimon, N.; Fallon, U.B.; O'Mahony, D.; Loftus, B.G.; Bury, G.; Murphy, A.W. & Kelleher, C.C.; Lifeways Cross Generation Cohort Study Steering Group. (2007). Mothers' dietary patterns during pregnancy and the risk of asthma symptoms in children at 3 years. *Irish Medical Journal*, Vol.100, No.8 suppl, (September 2007), pp. 27-32.

Funaguchi, N.; Ohno, Y.; La, B.L.; Asai, T.; Yuhgetsu, H.; Sawada, M.; Takemura, G.; Minatoguchi, S.; Fujiwara, T. & Fujiwara, H. (2007). Narirutin inhibits airway inflammation in an allergic mouse model. *Clinical and Experimental Pharmacology and Physiology*, Vol.34, No.8, (August 2007), pp. 766-770.

Garcia-Marcos, L.; Canflanca, I.M.; Garrido, J.B.; Varela, A.L.; Garcia-Hernandez, G.; Guillen Grim, F.; Gonzalez-Diaz, C.; Carvajal-Uruena, I.; Arnedo-Pena, A.; Busquets-Monge, R.M.; Morales Suarez-Varela, M. & Blanco-Quiros, A. (2007). Relationship of asthma and rhinoconjunctivitis with obesity, exercise and Mediterranean diet in Spanish schoolchildren. *Thorax*, Vol.62, No.6, (June 2007), pp. 503-508.

Garcia, V.; Arts, I.C.; Sterne, J.A.; Thompson, R.L. & Shaheen, S.O. (2005). Dietary intake of flavonoids and asthma in adults. *European Respiratory Journal*, Vol.26, No.3, (September 2005), pp. 449-452.

Gauchat, J.F.; Henchoz, S.; Mazzei, G.; Aubry, J.P.; Brunner, T.; Blasey, H.; Life, P.; Talabot, D.; Flores-Romo, L.; Thompson J.; Kishi, K.; Butterfield, J.; Dahinden, C. & Bonnefoy, J.Y. (1993). Induction of human IgE synthesis in B cells by mast cells and basophils. *Nature*, Vol.365, No.6444, (September 1993), pp. 340-343.

Gong, J.H.; Shin, D.; Han, S.Y.; Kim, J.L. & Kang, Y.H. (2012). Kaempferol suppresses eosinophil infiltration and airway inflammation in airway epithelial cells and in mice with allergic asthma. *The Journal of Nutrition*, Vol.142, No.1, (January 2012), pp. 47-56.

Grammatikos, A.P. (2008). The genetic and environmental basis of atopic diseases. *Annals of Medicine*, Vol.40, No.7, (September 2008), pp. 482-495.

Greiner, A.N.; Hellings, P.W.; Rotiroti, G. & Scadding, G.K. (2011). Allergic rhinitis. *Lancet*, Vol.378, No.9809, (December 2011), pp. 2112-2122.

Gry, J.; Black, L.; Eriksen, F.D.; Pilegaard, K.; Plumb, J.; Plumb, J.; Rhodes, M.; Sheehan, D.; Kiely, M. & Kroon, P.A. (2007). EuroFIR-BASIS – a combined composition and biological activity database for bioactive compounds in plant-based foods. *Trends in Food Science & Technology*, Vol.18, No.8, (August 2007), pp. 434-444.

Harborne, J.B. & Williams, C.A. (2000). Advances in flavonoid research since 1992. *Phytochemistry*, Vol.55, No.6, (November 2000), pp. 481-504.

Higa, S.; Hirano, T.; Kotani, M.; Matsumoto, M.; Fujita, A.; Suemura, M.; Kawase, I. & Tanaka, T. (2003). Fisetin, a flavonol, inhibits TH2-type cytokine production by activated human basophils. *Journal of Allergy and Clinical Immunology*, Vol.111, No.6, (June 2003), pp. 1299-1306.

Hirano, T.; Higa, S.; Arimitsu, J.; Naka, T.; Shima, Y.; Ohshima, S.; Fujimoto, M.; Yamadori, T.; Kawase, I. & Tanaka, T. (2004). Flavonoids such as luteolin, fisetin and apigenin are inhibitors of interleukin-4 and interleukin-13 production by activated human basophils. *International Archives of Allergy and Immunology*, Vol.134, No.2, (June 2004), pp. 135-140.

Hirano, T.; Arimitsu, J.; Higa, S.; Naka, T.; Ogata, A.; Shima, Y.; Fujimoto, M.; Yamadori, T.; Ohkawara, T.; Kuwahara, Y.; Kawai, M.; Kawase, I. & Tanaka, T. (2006). Luteolin, a flavonoid, inhibits CD40 ligand expression by activated human basophils. *International Archives of Allergy and Immunology*, Vol.140, No.2, (April 2006), pp. 150-156.

Hirano, T.; Kawai, M.; Arimitsu, J.; Ogawa, M.; Kuwahara, Y.; Hagihara, K.; Shima, Y.; Narazaki, M.; Ogata, A.; Koyanagi, M.; Kai, T.; Shimizu, R.; Moriwaki, M.; Suzuki, Y.; Ogino, S.; Kawase, I. & Tanaka, T. (2009). Preventative effect of a flavonoid, enzymatically modified isoquercitrin on ocular symptoms of Japanese cedar pollinosis. *Allergology International*, Vol.58, No.3, (September 2009), pp. 373-382.

Ho, S.M. (2010). Environmental epigenetics of asthma: an update. *Journal of Allergy and Clinical Immunology*, Vol.126, No.3, (September 2010), pp. 453-465.

Holgate, S.T. (1999). The epidemic of allergy and asthma. *Nature*, Vol.402, No.6760 Suppl, (November 1999), pp. B2-4.

Hollman, P.C. & Katan, M.B. (1999). Dietary flavonoids: intake, health effects and bioavailability. *Food & Chemical Toxicology*, Vol.37, No.9-10, (September-October 1999), pp. 937-942.

Horiguchi, S. & Saito, Y. (1964). Discovery of Japanese cedar pollinosis in Nikko, Ibaraki prefecture. *Arerugi*, Vol.13, (January-February 1964), pp. 16-18.

Jiang, J.S.; Chien, H.C.; Chen, C.M.; Lin, C.N. & Ko, W.C. (2007). Potent suppressive effects of 3-*O*-methylquercetin 5,7,3′,4′-*O*-tetraacetate on ovalbumin-induced airway hyperresponsiveness. *Planta Medica*, Vol.73, No.11, (September 2007), pp. 1156-1162.

Jung, C.H.; Lee, J.Y.; Cho, C.H. & Kim, C.J. (2007). Anti-asthmatic action of quercetin and rutin in conscious guinea-pigs challenged with aerosolized ovalbumin. *Archives of Pharmacal Research*, Vol.30, No.12, (December 2007), pp. 1599-1607.

Kaneko, Y.; Motohashi, Y.; Nakamura, H.; Endo, T. & Eboshiba, A. (2005). Increasing prevalence of Japanese cedar pollinosis: a meta-regression analysis. *International Archives of Allergy and Immunology*, Vol.136, No.4, (April 2005), pp. 365-371.

Kawai, M.; Hirano, T.; Higa, S.; Arimitsu, J.; Maruta, M.; Kuwahara, Y.; Ohkawara, T.; Hagihara, K.; Yamadori, T.; Shima, Y.; Ogata, A.; Kawase, I. & Tanaka, T. (2007). Flavonoids and related compounds as anti-allergic substances. *Allergology International*, Vol.56, No.2, (June 2007), pp. 113-123.

Kawai, M.; Hirano, T.; Arimitsu, J.; Higa, S.; Kuwahara, Y.; Hagihara, K.; Shima, Y.; Narazaki, M.; Ogata, A.; Koyanagi, M.; Kai, T.; Shimizu, R.; Moriwaki, M.; Suzuki, Y.; Ogino, S.; Kawase, I. & Tanaka, T. (2009). Enzymatically modified isoquercitrin, a flavonoid, on symptoms of Japanese cedar pollinosis: a randomized double-blind placebo-controlled trial. *International Archives of Allergy and Immunology*, Vol.149, No.4, (July 2009), pp. 359-368.

Kim, S.H.; Kim, B.K. & Lee, Y.C. (2011). Antiasthmatic effects of hesperdin, a potential Th2 cytokine antagonist, in a mouse model of allergic asthma. *Mediators of Inflammation*, (May 2011), 2011;485402.

Kimata, M.; Shichijo, M.; Miura, T.; Serizawa, I.; Inagaki, N. & Nagai, H. (2000a). Effects of luteolin, quercetin and baicalein on immunoglobulin E-mediated mediator release from human cultured mast cells. *Clinical & Experimental Allergy*, Vol.30, No.4, (April 2000), pp. 501-508.

Kimata, M.; Inagaki, N. & Nagai, H. (2000b). Effects of luteolin and other flavonoids on IgE-mediated allergic reactions. *Plant Medicine*, Vol.66, No.1, (February 2000), pp. 25-29.

Kishi, K.; Saito, M.; Saito, T.; Kumemura, M.; Okamatsu, H.; Okita, M. & Takazawa, K. (2005). Clinical efficacy of apple polyphenol for treating cedar pollinosis. *Bioscience, Biotechnology, and Biochemistry*, Vol.69, No.4, (April 2005), pp. 829-832.

Knekt, P.; Kumpulainen, J.; Jarvinen, R.; Rissanen, H.; Heliovaara, M.; Reunanen, A.; Hakulinen, T. & Aromaa A. (2002). Flavonoid intake and risk of chronic diseases. *The American Journal of Clinical Nutrition*, Vol.76, No.3, (September 2002), pp. 560-568.

Kotani, M.: Matsumoto, M.; Fujita, A.; Higa, S.; Wang, W.; Suemura, M.; Kishimoto, T. & Tanaka, T. (2000). Persimmon leaf extract and astragalin inhibit development of dermatitis and IgE elevation in NC/Nga mice. *Journal of Allergy and Clinical Immunology*, Vol.106(1 Pt 1), (July 2000), pp. 159-166.

Kouda, K.; Tanaka, T.; Kouda, M.; Takeuchi, H.; Takeuchi, A.; Nakamura, H. & Takigawa, M. (2000). Low-energy diet in atopic dermatitis patients: clinical findings and DNA damage. *Journal of Physiological Anthropology and Applied Human Science*, Vol.19, No.5, (September 2000), pp. 225-228.

Kozyrskyj, A.L.; Bahreinian, S. & Azad, M.B. (2011). Early life exposures: impact on asthma and allergic disease. *Current Opinion in Allergy and Clinical Immunology*, Vol.11, No.5, (October 2011). pp. 400-406.

La Vecchia, C.; Decarli, A. & Pagano, R. (1998). Vegetable consumption and risk of chronic disease. *Epidemiology*, Vol.9, No.2, (March 1998), pp. 208-210.

Lee, T.P.; Matteliano, M.L. & Middleton, E.J. (1982). Effect of quercetin on human polymorphonuclear leukocyte lysosomal enzyme release and phospholipid metabolism. *Life Sciences*, Vol.31, No.24, (December 1982), pp. 2765-2774.

Leemans, J.; Cambier, C.; Chandler, T.; Billen, F.; Clercx, C.; Kirschvink, N. & Gustin, P. (2010). Prophylactic effects of omega-3 polyunsaturated fatty acids and luteolin on airway hyperresponsiveness and inflammation in cats with experimentally-induced asthma. *The Veterinary Journal*, Vol.184, No.1, (April 2010), pp. 111-114.

Li, R.R.; Pang, L.L.; Du, Q.; Shi, Y.; Dai, W.J. & Yin, K.S. (2010). Apigenin inhibits allergen-induced airway inflammation and switches immune response in a murine model of asthma. *Immunopharmacology and Immunotoxicology*, Vol.32, No.3, (September 2010), pp. 364-370.

Maeda-Yamamoto, M.; Ema, K.; Monobe, M.; Shibuichi, I.; Shinoda, Y.; Yamamoto, T. & Fujisawa, T. (2009). The efficacy of early treatment of seasonal allergic rhinitis with benifuuki green tea containing *O*-methylated catechin before pollen exposure: an open randomized study. *Allergology International*, Vol.58, No.3, (September 2009), pp. 437-444.

Makino, T.; Furuta, Y.; Fujii, H.; Nakagawa, T.; Wakushima, H.; Saito, K. & Kano, Y. (2001). Effect of oral treatment of Perilla frutescens and its constituents on type-1 allergy in mice. *Biological and Pharmaceutical Bulletin*, Vol.24, No.10, (October 2001), pp. 1206-1209.

Manach, C.; Scalbert, A.; Morand, C.; Remesy, C.; Jimenez, L. (2004). Polyphenols: food sources and bioavailability. *The American Journal of Clinical Nutrition*, Vol.79, No.5, (May 2004), pp. 727-747.

Marshall, N.B. & Kerkvliet, N.I. (2010). Dioxin and immune regulation: emerging role of aryl hydrocarbon receptor in the generation of regulatory T cells. *Annals of the New York Academy of Sciences*, Vol.1183, (January 2010), pp. 25-37.

Matsuda, H.; Watanabe, N.; Geba, G.P.; Sperl, J.; Tsudzuki, M.; Hiroi, J.; Matsumoto, M.; Ushio, H.; Saito, S.; Askenase, P.W. & Ra, C. (1997). Development of atopic dermatitis-like skin lesion with IgE hyperproduction in NC/Nga mice. *International Immunology*, Vol.9, No.3, (May 1997), pp. 461-466.

Matsumoto, M.; Kotani, M.; Fujita, A.; Higa, S.; Kishimoto, T.; Suemura, M. & Tanaka, T. (2002). Oral administration of persimmon leaf extract ameliorates skin symptoms and transepidermal water loss in atopic dermatitis model mice, NC/Nga. *British Journal of Dermatology*, Vol.146, No.2, (February 2002), pp. 221-227.

McKeever, T.M. & Britton, J. (2004). Diet and asthma. *American Journal of Respiratory Critical Care of Medicine*, Vol.170, No.7, (October 2004), pp. 725-729.

Middleton, E.J.; Drzewiecki, G. & Krishnarao, D. (1981). Quercetin: an inhibitor of antigen-induced human basophil histamine release. *The Journal of Immunology*, Vol.127, No.2, (August 1981), pp. 546-550.

Middleton, E.J. & Kandaswami, C. (1992). Effects of flavonoids on immune and inflammatory cell functions. *Biochemical Pharmacology*, Vol.43, No.6, (March 1992), pp. 1167-1179.

Middleton, E.J.; Kandaswari, C. & Theoharides, T.C. (2000). The effects of plant flavonoids on mammalian cells: implications for inflammation, heart disease, and cancer. *Pharmacological Reviews*, Vol.52, No.4, (December 2000), pp. 673-751.

Neveu, V.; Perez-Jimenez, J.; Vos, F.; Crespy, V.; Du Chaffaut, L.; Mennen, L.; Knox, C.; Eisner, R.; Cruz, J.; Wishart, D. & Scalbert, A. (2010). Phenol-Explorer: an online comprehensive database on polyphenol contents in foods. *Database (Oxford)*, 2010;2010:bap024.

Nolte, H.; Backer, V. & Porsbjerg, C. (2001). Environmental factors as a cause for the increase in allergic disease. *Annals of Allergy, Asthma & Immunology*, Vol.87(6 Suppl 3), (December 2001), pp. 7-11.

Nurmatov, U.; Devereux, G. & Sheikh, A. (2011). Nutrients and foods for the primary prevention of asthma and allergy: systemic review and meta-analysis. *Journal of Allergy and Clinical Immunology*, Vol.127, No.3, (March 2011), pp. 724-733.

Okamaoto, Y.; Horiguchi, S.; Yamamoto, H.; Yonekura, S. & Hanazawa T. (2009). Present situation of cedar pollinosis in Japan and its immune responses. *Allergology International*, Vol.58, No.2, (March 2009), pp. 155-162.

Oku, H. & Ishiguro, K. (2001). Antipruritic and antidermatitic effects of extract and compounds of *Impatiens balsamina* L. in atopic dermatitis model NC mice. *Phytotherapy Research*, Vol.15, No.6, (September 2001), pp. 506-510.

Ozdoganoglu, T. & Songu, M. (2012). The burden of allergic rhinitis and asthma. *Therapeutic Advances in Respiratory Disease*, Vol.6, No.1, (January 2012), pp. 11-23.

Park, H.J.; Lee, C.M.; Jung, I.D.; Lee, J.S.; Jeong, Y.I.; Chang, J.H.; Chun, S.H.; Kim, M.J.; Choi, I.W.; Ahn, S.C.; Shin, Y.K.; Yeom, S.R. & Park, Y.M. (2009). Quercetin regulates Th1/Th2 balance in a murine model of asthma. *International Immunopharmacology*, Vol.9, No.3, (March 2009), pp. 261-267.

Perez-Jimenez, J.; Neveu, V.; Vos, F. & Scalbert, A. (2010). Systematic analysis of the content of 502 polyphenols in 452 foods and beverages: an application of the Phenol-Explorer database. *Journal of Agricultural and Food Chemistry*, Vol.58, No.8, (April 2010), pp. 4959-4969.

Perez-Jimenez, J.; Fezeu, L.; Touvier, M.; Arnault, N.; Manach, C.; Hercberg, S.; Galan, P. & Scalbert, A. (2011). Dietary intake of 337 polyphenols in French adults. *The American Journal of Clinical Nutrition*, Vol.93, No.6, (June 2011), pp. 1220-1228.

Rogerio, A.P.; Kanashiro, A.; Fontanari, C.; da Silva, E.V.; Lucisano-Valim, Y.M.; Soares, E.G. & Faccioli, L.H. (2007). Anti-inflammatory activity of quercetin and isoquercitrin in experimental murine allergic asthma. *Inflammation Research*, Vol.56, No.10, (October 2007), pp. 402-408.

Rosenwasser, L.J. (2011). Mechanisms of IgE inflammation. *Current Allergy and Asthma Reports*, Vol.11, No.2, (April 2011), pp. 178-183.

Russo, M.; Spagnuolo, C.; Tedesco, I.; Bilotto, S. & Russo, G.L. (2012). The flavonoid quercetin in disease prevention and therapy: facts and fancies. *Biochemical Pharmacology*, Vol.83, No.1, (January 2012), pp. 6-15.

Salim, E.I.; Kaneko, M.; Wanibuchi, H.; Morimura, K. & Fukushima, S. (2004). Lack of carcinogenicity of enzymatically modified isoquercitrin in F344/DuCrj rats. *Food and Chemical Toxicology*, Vol.42, No.12, (December 2004), pp. 1949-1969.

Sealbert, A.; Manach, C.; Morand, C.; Remesy, C. & Jimenez, L. (2005). Dietary polyphenols and the prevention of diseases. *Critical Reviews in Food Science and Nutrition*, Vol.45, No.4, (April 2005), pp. 287-306.

Segawa, S.; Takata, Y.; Wakita, Y.; Kaneko, T.; Kaneda, H.; Watari, J.; Enomoto, T. & Enomoto, T. (2007). Clinical effects of a hop water extract on Japanese cedar pollinosis during the pollen season: a double-blind, placebo-controlled trial. *Bioscience, Biotechnology, and Biochemistry*, Vol.71, No.8, (October 2007), pp. 1955-1962.

Shaheen, S.O.; Sterne, J.A.; Thompson, R.L.; Songhurst, C.E.; Margetts, B.M. & Burney, P.G. (2001). Dietary antioxidants and asthma in adults: population-based case-control study. *American Journal of Respiratory and Critical Care Medicine*, Vol.164(10 Pt 1), pp. 1823-1828.

Shishebor, F.; Behroo, L.; Ghafouriyan Broujerdnia, M.; Namjoyan, F. & Latifi, S.M. (2010). Quercetin effectively quells peanut-induced anaphylactic reactions in the peanut sensitized rats. *Iranian Journal of Allergy, Asthma and Immunology*, Vol.9, No.1, (March 2010), pp 27-34.

Singh, A.; Holvoet, A. & Mercenier, A. (2011). Dietary polyphenols in the prevention and treatment of allergic diseases. *Clinical & Experimental Allergy*, Vol.41, No.10, (October 2011), pp. 1346-1359.

Song, M.Y.; Jeong, G.S.; Lee, H.S.; Kwon, K.S.; Lee, S.M.; Park, J.W.; Kim, Y.C. & Park, B.H. (2010). Sulfuretin attenuates allergic airway inflammation in mice. *Biochemical and Biophysical Research Communications*, Vol.400, No.1, (September 2010). pp. 83-88.

Stone, K.D.; Prussin, C. & Metcalfe, D.D. (2010). IgE, mast cells, basophils, and eosinophils. *Journal of Allergy and Clinical Immunology*, Vol.125(2 Suppl 2), (February 2010), pp. S73-80.

Takano, H.; Osakabe, N.; Sanbongi, C.; Yanagisawa, R.; Inoue, K.; Yasuda, A.; Natsume, M.; Baba, S.; Ichiishi, E. & Yoshikawa, T. (2004). Extract of Perilla frutescens enriched for rosmarinic acid, a polyphenolic phytochemical, inhibits seasonal allergic rhinoconjunctivitis in humans. *Experimental Biology and Medicine*, Vol.229, No.3, (March 2004), pp. 247-254.

Tamay, Z.; Akcay, A.; Ones, U.; Guler, N.; Kilic, G. & Zencir, M. (2007). Prevalence and risk factors for allergic rhinitis in primary school children. *International Journal of Pediatric Otorhinolaryngology*, Vol.71, No.3, (March 2007), pp. 463-471.

Tanaka, T.; Kouda, K.; Kotani, M.; Takeuchi, A.; Tabei, T.; Masamoto, Y.; Nakamura, H.; Takigawa, M.; Suemura, M.; Takeuchi, H. & Kouda, M. (2001). Vegetarian diet ameliorates symptoms of atopic dermatitis through reduction of the number of peripheral eosinophils and of PGE2 synthesis by monocytes. *Journal of Physiological Anthropology and Applied Human Science*, Vol.20, No.6, (November 2001), pp. 353-361.

Tanaka, T.; Higa, S.; Hirano, T.; Kotani, M.; Matsumoto, M.; Fujita, A. & Kawase, I. (2003). Flavonoids as potential anti-allergic substances. *Current Medicinal Chemistry-Anti-Inflammatory & Anti-Allergy Agents*, Vol.2, No.1, (March 2003), pp. 57-65.

Tanaka, T.; Higa, S.; Hirano, T.; Arimitsu, J.; Naka, T.; Shima, Y.; Ohshima, S.; Fujimoto, M.; Yamadori, T. & Kawase, I. (2004). Is an appropriate intake of flavonoids a prophylactic means or complementary and alternative medicine for allergic diseases? *Recent Research Developmental Allergy & Clinical Immunology*, Vol.5, (February 2004), pp. 1-14.

Tanaka, T.; Hirano, T.; Kawai, M.; Arimistu, J.; Hagihara, K.; Ogawa, M.; Kuwahara, Y.; Shima, Y.; Narazaki, M.; Ogata, A. & Kawase, I. (2011). Flavonoids, natural inhibitors of basophil activation. Paul, K. Vellis, (ed.), *Basophil Granulocytes,* Nova Science Publishers, Inc., New York, 2011; Chapter 4, pp 61-72.

USDA database for the flavonoid content of selective foods. Release 3. (2011). Prepared by Seema Bhagwat, David B. Haytowitz and Joanne M. Holden. U.S. Department of Agriculture. (September 2011), URL: *http://www.ars.usda.gov/nutrientdata*

Visioli, F.; De La Lastra, C.A.; Andres-Lacueva, C.; Aviram, M.; Calhau, C.; Cassano, A.; D'Archivio, M.; Faria, A.; Fave, G.; Fogliano, V.; Llorach, R.; Vitaglione, P.; Zoratti, M. & Edeas, M. (2011). Polyphenols and human health: a prospectus. *Critical Reviews in Food Sciences and Nutrition*, Vol.51, No.6, (July 2011), pp. 524-546.

Willers, S.M.; Devereux, G.; Craig, L.C.; McNeill, G.; Wijga, A.H.; Abou, El-Magd, W.; Turner, S.W.; Helms, P.J. & Seaton, A. (2007). Maternal food consumption during pregnancy and asthma, respiratory and atopic symptoms in 5-year-old children. *Thorax*, Vol.62, No.9, (September 2007), pp. 773-779.

Williams, C.A. & Grayer, R.J. (2004). Anthocyanins and other flavonoids. *Natural Product Reports*, Vol.21, No.4, (August 2004), pp. 539-573.

Wilson, D.; Evans, M.; Guthrie, N.; Sharma, P.; Baisley, J.; Schonlau, F. & Burki, C. (2010). A randomized, double-blind, placebo-controlled exploratory study to evaluate the potential of pycnogenol for improving allergic rhinitis symptoms. *Phytotherapy Research*, Vol.24, No.8, (August 2010), pp. 1115-1119.

Wu, M.Y.; Hung, S.K. & Fu, S.L. (2011). Immunosuppressive effects of fisetin in ovalbumin-induced asthma through inhibition of NF-kB activity. *Journal of Agricultural and Food Chemistry*, Vol.59, No.19, (October 2011), pp. 10496-10504.

Wu, Y.Q.; Zhou, C.H.; Tao, J. & Li, S.N. (2006). Antagonistic effects of nobiletin, a polymethoxyflavonoid, on eosinophilic airway inflammation of asthmatic rats and relevant mechanisms. *Life Sciences*, Vol.78, No.23, (May 2006), pp. 2689-2696.

Yano, S.; Umeda, D.; Yamashita, S.; Ninomiya, Y.; Sumida, M.; Fujimura, Y.; Yamada, K. & Tachibana, H. (2007). Dietary flavones suppress IgE and Th2 cytokines in OVA-immunized BALB/c mice. *European Journal of Nutrition*, Vol.46, No.5, (August 2007), pp. 257-263.

Yano, S.; Umeda, D.; Yamashita, S.; Yamada, K. & Tachibana, H. (2009). Dietary apigenin attenuates the development of atopic dermatitis-like skin lesions in NC/Nga mice. *The Journal of Nutritional Biochemistry*, Vol.20, No.11, (November 2009), pp. 876-881.

Yoshimoto, T.; Furukawa, M.; Yamamoto, S.; Horie, T. & Watanabe-Kohno, S. (1983). Flavonoids: potent inhibitors of arachidonate 5-lipoxygenase. *Biochemical and Biophysical Research Communications*, Vol.116, No.2, (October 1983), pp. 612-618.

Yoshimura, M.; Enomoto, T.; Dake, Y.; Okuno, Y.; Ikeda, H.; Cheng, L. & Obata, A (2007). An evaluation of the clinical efficacy of tomato extract for perennial allergic rhinitis. *Allergology International*, Vol.56, Vol.3, (September 2007), pp. 225-230.

Yun, M.Y.; Yang, J.H.; Kim, D.K.; Cheong, K.J.; Song, H.H.; Kim, D.H.; Cheong, K.J.; Kim, Y.I. & Shin, S.C. (2010). Therapeutic effects of Baicalein on atopic dermatitis-like skin lesions of NC/Nga mice induced by dermatophagoides pteronyssinus. *International Immunopharmacology*, Vol.10, No.9, (September 2010), pp. 1142-1148.